W9-CWV-985

PHYSICIAN-PATIENT COMMUNICATION

PHYSICIAN-PATIENT COMMUNICATION

Readings and Recommendations

Edited by

GEORGE HENDERSON, Ph.D.

S.N. Goldman Professor of Human Relations
Professor of Education and Associate Professor of Sociology
University of Oklahoma
Norman, Oklahoma

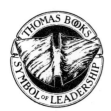

CHARLES C THOMAS · PUBLISHER
Springfield · Illinois · U.S.A.

WILLIAM MADISON RANDALL LIBRARY UNC AT WILMINGTON

Published and Distributed Throughout the World by
CHARLES C THOMAS • PUBLISHER
Bannerstone House
301-327 East Lawrence Avenue, Springfield, Illinois, U.S.A.

This book is protected by copyright. No part of it
may be reproduced in any manner without written
permission from the publisher.

© *1981, by* CHARLES C THOMAS • PUBLISHER
ISBN 0-398-04447-3
Library of Congress Catalog Card Number: 80-39742

With THOMAS BOOKS careful attention is given to all details of manufacturing and design. It is the Publisher's desire to present books that are satisfactory as to their physical qualities and artistic possibilities and appropriate for their particular use. THOMAS BOOKS will be true to those laws of quality that assure a good name and good will.

Library of Congress Cataloging in Publication Data
Main entry under title

Physician-patient communication.

   Includes bibliographies and index.
   1. Physician and patient—Addresses, essays, lectures. 2. Interpersonal communication—Addresses, essays, lectures. I. Henderson, George, 1932-   [DNLM: 1. Physician-patient relations. 2. Communication.   W 62 P578]
R727.3.P48   610.69'6   80-39742
ISBN 0-398-04465-1

Printed in the United States of America
PS-R-1

R 727
3
.P48

CONTRIBUTORS

K. BIRKINSHAW, M.B., B.S., F.F.A.R.C.S. Consultant Anaesthetist, Bronglais General Hospital, Great Britain

DAN BLAZER, M.D., M.P.H. Associate Professor of Psychiatry
and Associate Director for Programs, Center for the Study of
Aging and Human Development, Duke University, Durham,
North Carolina

JOHN G. BRUHN, Ph.D. Dean, School of Allied Health
Sciences, University of Texas Medical Branch, Galveston

RACHEL DeVRIES, R.N. Former Nurse Chairman, Baltimore
Cancer Research Program, National Cancer Institute, Baltimore, Maryland

VICTOR M. SANTANA CARLOS, M.D. Centro de Medicina de
Rebalitacão, Alcoitão-Estoril, Portugal

D.M. GRENNAN, M.D., Ph.D., M.R.C.P. Senior Lecturer,
Department of Medicine, University of Otago Medical School,
Dunedin, New Zealand

ANNE P. HAHN, M.S.W. Head, Social Work Section, Baltimore
Cancer Research Program, National Cancer Institute, Baltimore, Maryland

GEORGE HENDERSON, Ph.D. S.N. Goldman Professor of
Human Relations, Professor of Education and Associate
Professor of Sociology, University of Oklahoma, Norman

BARBARA M. KORSCH, M.D. Patient-Care Coordinator, Childrens Hospital, Los Angeles, California

HARRY KROP, Ph.D. Psychology Services, Veterans Administration Hospital, Gainesville, Florida

AUSTIN H. KUTSCHER, Ph.D. Professor, Columbia University, Presbyterian Medical Center, New York, New York

MICHAEL McLANE, M.A. Psychology Service, Veterans Administration Hospital, Gainesville, Florida

CHRISTINE McNAMEE, R.N., B.Sc.N. Instructor, St. Paul's
Hospital School of Nursing, Vancouver, British Columbia,
Canada

v

219877

JAWAHAR MEHTA, M.D. Associate Professor of Cardiovascular Medicine, University of Florida Department of Medicine, Gainesville

VIDA FRANCIS NEGRETE, M.S. Research Associate, Childrens Hospital, Los Angeles, California

D.G. PALMER, M.D., M.R.C.P., F.R.A.C.P. Associate Professor, Department of Medicine, University of Otago Medical School, Dundein, New Zealand

NATHAN SCHNAPER, M.D., F.A.P.A., F.A.C.P. Chief, Psychiatry Section, Baltimore Cancer Research Program, National Cancer Institute, Professor of Psychiatry, School of Medicine, University of Maryland, Baltimore

ROGER W. SHUY, Ph.D. Senior Linguist, Center for Applied Linguistics, Washington, D.C.

STEPHEN M. SOREFF, M.D. Director of Emergency and Consultation Psychiatry, Maine Medical Center, Portland

SUSAN TAYLOR Department of Pharmacy, University of Otago, Dundein, New Zealand

JON R. WEINBERG, Ph.D. Psychologist, Meadowbrook Treatment Center; Director of Education and Training, the Hennepin County Alcoholism and Inebriety Program, Minneapolis, Minnesota

THOMAS WOLMAN, M.D. Instructor in Psychiatry, Thomas Jefferson University School of Medicine; Staff Psychiatrist, Jefferson Community Mental Health Center, Philadelphia, Pennsylvania

PREFACE

It is becoming increasingly clear that in order to be optimally effective as care providers physicians must possess interpersonal communication skills. Even so, numerous physicians have lamented the failure of their former teachers to expose them to human relations concepts and techniques needed to help diverse patient populations. No student should graduate from medical school without learning basic physician-patient communication skills.

In order to compile a helpful text focusing mainly on physician-patient communication, I have elected to draw upon the expertise of several persons. There are some obvious short-comings in books of readings, especially uneven writing styles. However, the readings format has made it possible for me to bring together in one text several multidisciplinary, international articles of considerable importance. The broad range of academic disciplines and medical specializations represented in this volume provide a valuable theoretical overview and practical clinical insight focusing on the physician-patient communication process.

But this is not a disparate collection of articles. Although each chapter is a complete unit, all of them are interrelated when read as a total package. Each was selected with two major criteria in mind: (1) clear presentation of the issues and (2) relevance. Topics discussed briefly in Chapter 1 are elaborated on in later chapters. In addition to presenting various theories and concepts of communication, the book includes strategies for conducting medical interviews and implementing a health plan. Specific communication strategies are offered for physicians treating elderly, hard-of-hearing, alcoholic, arthritic, spinal cord injured, cardiac, hypertensive, and cancer patients. Because of their special nature, three chapters are devoted to communicating with dying patients and their relatives. Ample references are provided for individuals who wish to explore specific issues or topics in greater detail.

By drawing upon the writings of physicians and other health related professionals, I intentionally present practical suggestions for readers who desire to improve their own communication skills. I have not included unrealistic, utopian concepts. Instead, I have built this book upon the insights, achievements, and recommendations of dedicated practitioners trying to humanize orthodox medicine. The timeliness and insightfulness of their contributions have already elevated some of them to lofty academic and professional heights. There is much here for medical students as well as experienced practitioners—physicians, psychiatrists, psychologists, nurses, and medical technicians.

I am grateful to the authors and publishers who have given me permission to reprint their materials. Special thanks go to my wife, Barbara. Her willingness to read the manuscript and recommend additions and deletions helped me to complete a much delayed project.

G.H.

CONTENTS

PHYSICIAN-PATIENT COMMUNICATION

Chapter 1

THE IMPORTANCE OF COMMUNICATION

GEORGE HENDERSON

"Most laymen would take clinical ability for granted and will not judge the physician in terms of his basic medical skills, which they assume he possesses merely because he is a physician. He will be judged and then trusted accordingly solely in terms of the following: The genuineness of his interest, the thoroughness of his approach to the problem, his personal warmth, understanding and compassion, and finally the degree of clarity with which he gives the patient insight into what is wrong and what must be done."[1]

There is a growing trend in medical schools to include more coursework focusing on communication skills. Slowly, there is forming an international awareness of the inadequacy of the largely technical approach characterizing most medical curricula. David E. Reiser captured a bit of this inadequacy when discussing his own medical education: "Suddenly I realized what I had done, how cut off and alienated I had become. I brooded about the experience for the rest of the night. I looked back to the times in recent months when I had been arrogant and emotionally cold. I had walked away from more than one cry for help. I had gone into medicine to help other people, but seemed to be fleeing more and more from human contact. I began to wonder if the changes were irreversible. Was I alone in this dilemma?"[2]

Reiser's dilemma is not unique. Countless other physicians are torn by the nagging, dehumanizing consequences of medical education. Medical schools continue to produce graduates who are technically competent but interpersonally inadequate. The tools of the trade—medical paraphernalia and more than 10,000 medical terms—do little to produce physicians who feel comfortable communicating with their patients. Even the clinical training process of "going on rounds" does little to improve interpersonal skills. In Reiser's words: "Every morning, a small drove of doctors gathers around the patient's bed and begins the ritual. The whole ceremony is often terrifying and incomprehensible to the patient, whose dignity and privacy are often needlessly compromised. It is no accident that we doctors tend to travel in packs. I think deep down many of us are afraid to spend time alone with our patients."[3]

Once this pattern of avoiding interpersonal contact and walling in personal feeling is established, it is difficult to alter. Prakash Burra and Alexander M. Bryans said it quite well: "This ignoring of the interpersonal dimension in medical care, and investing heavily in the care-giver being technically competent and efficient, would seem to take its toll not only on the patient but also on the doctor himself."[4]

It should be made clear at the outset that I do not consider basic research and medical technology unimportant. On the contrary, without them orthodox medicine would be less than a science. However, I do not believe that patients should be treated as faceless human beings with interchangeable parts and nonrelevant cultural backgrounds. Neither do most physicians believe this.

DEFINITIONS OF COMMUNICATION

Broadly speaking, communication can be defined as a process by which a person sends a message—verbal or nonverbal or behavioral stimuli to someone else with the conscious intent of evoking a response. However, communication is neither static nor a thing. The key concept is "process." "It is a dynamic, circular process," David K. Berlo wrote: "We view events and relationships as dynamic, ever-changing, continuous."[5] As a continuous process, communication does not have a beginning, an end, or a fixed sequence. And since it is not static, communication is always moving. The various elements of the process are interrelated; each affects the others.

Effective communication refers to the process in which the

receiver interprets the message the same way intended by the sender. Donald W. Johnson listed seven basic elements of interpersonal communication:

1. The intentions, ideas, feelings of the sender and the behavior he selects to engage in, all of which leads to his sending a message which conveys some content.
2. The sender encoding his message by translating his ideas, feelings, and intentions into a message appropriate for transmission.
3. The transmission of the message to a receiver.
4. The channel through which the message is translated.
5. The receiver decoding the message by taking the stimuli received and interpreting their meaning. The interpretation of a message depends upon the receiver's comprehension of the content of the message and the intentions of the sender.
6. The receiver responding internally to his interpretation of the message.
7. The amount of noise in the above steps. Noise is any element that interferes with the communication process. In the sender, noise can refer to such things as the attitudes, prejudices, or frame of reference of the sender and the inappropriateness of his language or other expression to the message. In the receiver, noise refers to the decoding process. In the channel, noise refers to environmental sounds such as static or traffic, speech problems such as stammering, annoying or distracting mannerisms such as a tendency to mumble, or other distractions. To a large extent, the success of communication is determined by the degree to which noise is overcome or controlled.[6]

Numerous researchers have concluded that the single most important element in interpersonal communication is *sender credibility*—the attitude the receiver of a message has toward the sender's trustworthiness. As noted earlier, most patients view health care providers as medical experts who have substantial knowledge of diseases, illness, and cures. Credibility gaps are created when medical practitioners do not project empathy, warmth, friendliness, and concern for patients and their families. There are five variables used to determine the effectiveness of communication and the credibility of the sender: Who? Says What? In Which Channel? To Whom? With What Effect?[7]

Dean C. Barnlund cautions us to remember that communication is complex, irreversible, and involves the total personality.[8] In summary, communication does not refer to only verbal, explicit messages. Rather, it includes, as Jurgen Ruesch and Gregory Bateson noted, "all those processes by which people influence one another . . . This definition is based upon the premise that all actions and events have communicative aspects, as soon as they are perceived by a human being; it implies, furthermore, that such perception changes the information which an individual possesses and therefore influences him."[9]

MODELS OF COMMUNICATION

There are several models of communication but we shall briefly review only three: Claude Shannon's mathematical model,[10] W. L. Schramm's human communication transition model,[11] and Berlo's SMCR (Source, Message, Channel, Receiver) model.[12]

Shannon's mathematical model is the prototype for several human communication models. Unfortunately, Shannon did not include feedback in his model, which follows (Figure 1-1).

Unlike one-way communication described by Shannon, two-way communication is slower but more accurate. Furthermore, two-way communication is disorderly and the participants risk changing their beliefs, values, and behavior. Besides, less effort is required to maintain the *status quo*. The difficulty of achieving accurate communication was penned by an anonymous writer: "I know that you believe you understood what you think I said, but I'm not sure you realize that what you heard is not what I said." Physicians must constantly ask themselves if they are communicating with patients to hear or see something that will confirm their prejudices or if they are communicating to find out what the patients feel, think, and value.

Schramm's model incorporates the basic components of human communication (Figure 1-2).

As can be seen in the following diagram, Berlo's model is the best for our purpose (Figure 1-3).

Constructive feedback is (1) descriptive rather than evaluative, (2) specific rather than general, (3) considerate of the needs of both the sender and receiver, (4) focused on behavior the receiver can do something about, (5) solicited rather than imposed, (6) properly timed, and (7) checked to insure clear communication.

Simply stated, any communication must have a sender, a message, content, channel of transmission, a receiver, and response. A physician may desire to communicate a message to patients, but if there is noise in the transmission, they will not

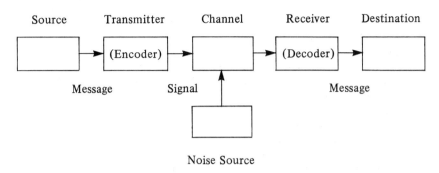

Figure 1-1

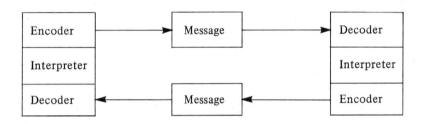

Figure 1-2

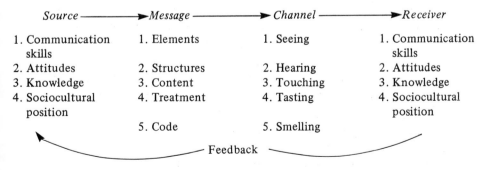

Figure 1-3

understand the message. Sometimes they will not even get the
message being sent.

> Habits of gesture-small movements of the hands, feet, face, eyes, nods,
> smiles, frown, fist shakes and a host of other common gestures-all
> communicate important understandings. For instance, the harried and
> brisk manner in which nurses and doctors enter and leave a patient's
> room often communicates to the patient that the staff is very busy and
> does not have much time to spend with patients or to meet their little
> needs and wants. Most patients are very sensitive to the mode in which
> care is provided. They look for willing and spontaneous treatment and
> service. They are alert and react quickly to facial expressions, tone of
> voice, and the general manner in which requests are received. They
> often interpret the smile of a physician or nurse as a sign that the
> hospital staff likes them and is willing to take care of them. On the
> other hand, a frown is sometimes seen as a sign of flat rejection.[13]

The results of ineffective communication ranges from low
patient morale to death. Thus effective communication is an
integral part of a physician's skill. A 1977 national survey noted
that 77 percent of 10,000 nurse respondents rated doctors less than
good in terms of their communication with patients.[14] Also in
1977, the University of North Carolina School of Public Health
released the results of a study focusing on patient failure to take
prescribed medication. The failure was positively correlated with
a breakdown of communication between physicians and patients.[15]

VERBAL COMMUNICATION

Verbal communication is the most important component of
physician-patient interaction. Verbal communication consists of
words uttered by individuals in an effort to transmit data, to solve
problems, or to merely acknowledge their own existence. Words
play a major part in our lives and therefore deserve considerable
scrutiny. The rookie police officer learns that words have the
power to transform seemingly lifeless and unrelated individuals
into a screaming, jeering, and destructive mob. In retrospect,
words have the power to mold thoughts, canalize feelings, and set
behavior in motion.

People of similar cultures agree that certain sounds, grunts,
and gibberings made with their tongues, teeth, throats, lungs,
and lips systematically stand for specified things or conditions.

All people utter sounds in hope that the persons who receive them will be in common agreement about their meaning. Indeed, words are what make us human; their value is transcendent. At the same time, words are full of human relations traps. Their meanings can be distorted and, when this occurs, a patient may experience physical pain and psychological misery beyond all reason. In extreme cases, patients' distortion of physicians' words have cost them their health and, in some cases, their lives.

There is no escape from this problem. Words are helpful, harmful, or neutral in their effect. To use an analogy, words are like a sharp ax—invaluable for cutting through barriers but also capable of injuring the people behind the barriers. For this reason, numerous writers have advised physicians that words and their meanings will, to a great extent, determine how successful or unsuccessful they will be in relating to their patients.

"The use of professional jargon is too often a major factor that inhibits effective communication, even when an attempt is made to develop good support. On the other hand, the use of precise dental and medical terms may be equally as confusing and alarming. The patient told that he has a lesion or a tumor, even when the term 'benign' is appended, may still come away with the idea that he has cancer. Simple terminology should be used and, if the patient does not understand, he should be given the opportunity to ask questions."[16]

Harry E. Munn, Jr. provides a helpful approach to determining whether a patient understands his/her diagnosis and the projected medical procedure. "Doctors and nurses should never ask patients, "Do you understand?" Munn advises. "In a sense this is calling for a predisposed answer and all the weight is on the patient to answer yes. Rather, we should explain the procedure and then ask, 'What do you understand?'"[17]

A general verbal climate of acceptance and warmth is more helpful than specific praise. Physicians who are insecure tend to hide behind their professional roles and jargon. Of course, the time available to converse with patients is not uniform. For example, generalists are able to spend more time with their patients than oral and maxillofacial surgeons. However, it is the quality—not the quantity—of the conversation that is important.

NONVERBAL COMMUNICATION

Nonverbal communication should never be considered an acceptable substitute for words unless the patient is deaf. Nonverbal communication is commonly called "body language." Technically, it is the science of *kinesics*. This science includes the study of reflexive and nonreflexive movements of a part or all of the body used by a person to communicate a message. There are several kinds of body language that physicians use, including the following.

GESTURES AND CLUSTERS OF GESTURES.   There are approximately 100,000 distinct gestures that have meaning to people around the world. These gestures are produced by facial expressions, postures, movements of the arms, hands, fingers, feet, legs, and so forth. Gestures are essential in face-to-face communication because they accentuate words.

MANNER OF SPEAKING.   The tone of an individual's voice, the placing of oral emphasis, is closely related to gestures. Specifically, the manner of speaking includes the quality, volume, pitch, and duration of speech. Relatedly, how a message is delivered will favorably or unfavorably influence the recipients.

ZONES OF TERRITORY.   Edward T. Hall coined the word "proxemics" to describe human zones of spatial territory and how they are used.[18] Zones of movement increase as intimacy decreases. That is, the more space available without other persons present, the more movement is likely to occur. In informal gatherings, a distance of six to eighteen inches is considered too close for the average American male, whereas this distance does not cause discomfort for the average American female. When our zones of territory are invaded or we in turn invade the territory of others we communicate our discomfort or apologize for our intrusion. The nature of medical work necessitates that physicians invade the intimate zones of patients—even when such an invasion is uncomfortable.

EYE CONTACT.   Most Americans are taught not to stare at other people. Instead they learn to acknowledge another person's presence through deliberate and polite inattention. That is, they look only long enough to make it clear that they see the other person and then look away. Through body language individuals conditioned to respond in this manner say, "I know you are here, but I will not intrude on your privacy or embarrass you with my stare." Physicians are taught to stare at patients—even if it embarrasses them.

TOUCHING. The sense of touch conveys acceptance or rejection, warmth or coldness, positive or negative feelings. Much of the physician's contact with patients require touching: "The touch of a doctor or nurse *can* be meaningful. Sensitive hands can be soothing to a patient, help relieve tension and fear, instill confidence and courage, and communicate understanding and a desire to help. One patient confided: 'The moment the doctor touched me, I was not afraid anymore. I knew I was going to be all right. It was in the touch. It was wonderful.'"[10] There are specific instances, such as the preservation of life, which require physicians to give little attention to the feelings of the person being touched and more attention to doing what is necessary to avert a loss or injury.

LISTENING. Effective communication does not occur unless effective listening also occurs. Medical interviews are designed to get and give information. It is during the interview that listening skills become crucial to diagnosis. In order to conduct a good interview, health care personnel must familiarize themselves with the purposes of specific interviews and methods of conducting effective interviews, including things to look for during the interview.

THE MEDICAL INTERVIEW

The major purpose of the medical interview is to collect historical information that can be used to make a diagnosis of disease and to understand the patient's illness. This, then, is the beginning of the relationship between a physician and his/her patient. While not a rigid order of data collection, the information obtained by the interviewer can be subsumed into five major categories:

1. *Present illness* is the recent health conditions that caused the patient to seek medical care.

2. *Past health* refers to the patient's general health, including illness and diagnosed diseases, prior to present illness.

3. *Family health* includes health histories of the patient's family, living and dead, with attention focused on possible

genetic and environmental sources of disease.

4. *Personal and social history* consists of sociopsychological life experiences that helped shape the patient's personality and physical health.

5. *Systems review* is the physician's summary of the body systems, with special attention given to symptoms not included in the patient's present illness or past health.

Information needed to complete each category seldom comes in the sequence listed above. Rather, information tends to flow from the patient in a free association, random thought manner. It is important for the interviewer to allow the patient to tell his/her medical story in a manner that is comfortable. As the information is obtained, it can be placed in the format of the medical history. Although all interviews do not follow the same course, the following steps are common:

1. The physician greets the patient, introduces himself/herself, and defines his/her professional role. Common courtesy dictates that the physician learns the patient's name and refers to it with proper title, e.g. Mr., Mrs., Miss, Dr., or Ms. When in doubt about how a patient prefers to be addressed, it is proper to ask, "How do you prefer that I address you, as 'Mrs. Smith' or 'Ms. Smith?'" The introduction usually is accompanied by a handshake. However, if the patient is too ill, placing a hand on the patient's hand or arm is suitable contact.

2. The physician inquires about how and what the patient is feeling at the moment. The first consideration should be to put the patient at ease and to make him/her as comfortable as possible. If available, the interview should be conducted in an unoccupied room or office. It is imperative that personal information is discussed in a setting as free as possible from eavesdroppers. Proper lighting, ventilation, and temperature are also components in putting the patient at ease. "How are you feeling?" is more than a social amenity; it should be a sincere invitation for the patient to self-disclose.

3. The physician encourages the patient to mention all symptoms and complaints leading to his/her current condition. This is best done when patients express themselves in their own words. It is during this phase that the physician has the first major opportunity to learn about the patient's personality and environmental influences.

4. The physician explores in greatest detail possible the etiology of the patient's current illness, including the sequence of each symptom. It is at this juncture that clues may develop that lead to past health, family history, and personal and social history.

5. The physician inquires about the patient's past health.

6. The physician inquires about the patient's family history. Past and current family member relationships with the patient may be important parts of the illness puzzle.

7. The physician inquires about the patient's current social life and past developments. The discussion of personal and social history, as well as details of past health and family health, are highly sensitive areas. Thus, this line of inquiry should be pursued when the patient has confidence in the physician. A statement such as "Do you mind talking about this?" is a way to allow the patient to delay the discussion until he/she feels ready. Each patient has the right to talk about specific issues in his/her own way and within his/her own timing.

8. The physician places the symptoms within regional and, if relevant, ethnic perspectives.

9. The physician checks the accuracy of all data and details collected to date and informs the patient of the next step. The physician should explain to the patient what records—if any— will be needed to assist in the data gathering.

Since the primary purpose of the interview is to elicit information about the patient's health, it is important to let the patient do most of the talking. The physician should direct the interview, but it should not be physician dominated. Self-expression on the part of the patient may uncover hidden illnesses, problems, and fears. There have been several studies of verbal interaction between physicians and patients.[20,21,22] D. J. G. Bain observed twenty-two family physicians over a period of one year and concluded (1) that physicians did more talking than patients and (2) the main thrust of the physicians' communication was to acquire facts, interpret symptoms and signs, and create a diagnostic label. On the other hand, their patients were more concerned with how the findings would affect social and family matters.[23]

The use of patient history questionnaires are time saving but often irritating to patients. The impersonal nature of questionnaires implies coldness, detachment, and invasion of privacy.

This is not to say that the data is not needed. Rather, I am saying that sometimes a less formal, more personal approach is needed before patients will feel good about filling out forms. For some patients, four words—"Tell me about yourself"—initially elicit more data than structured questions.

> It is almost impossible to touch on this subject without inveighing Sir William Osler's plea to "listen to the patient." It is old, and in spite of the overwhelming array of technology we have available, that admonition is no less true today than then. Indeed, since so many aggressive and invasive procedures are available, with huge potentials for both help and harm, the art of listening and communicating has become even more important. In Sir William's day, physicians were often unable to change the course of a disease, so that much of the time accurate diagnosis was an academic exercise. Not so now. A patient's personal history should be utilized to the fullest, so that when combined with objectivity, a reasonable assessment can be drawn, and a rational plan as to treatment can be developed. Otherwise, the initial management of a patient's illness may be inadequate, with the cost measured in both time and money and possible morbidity related to unnecessary diagnostic or therapeutic adventures.[24]

Refusing to acknowledge their own ineffective communication skills, many physicians label patients "poor historians." Through their own ineptness, these physicians greatly diminish or even destroy their patients' ability to present helpful histories. Who, we might ask, are the poor historians in this instance—patients or physicians?

PHYSICIAN DILEMMAS

The collective attempt of the human race to understand its existence is a classical study in frustration. *Homo sapiens* have always been concerned with structuring universal reality, not only temporarily but ultimately. Our confrontations with the universe arouse complex emotions within us. That is, most people are puzzled by cyclic patterns of the seasons, the unerring polarities of days and nights, the conflict between reason and emotion, the glorious process of birth, and the inevitable call of death. In short, human life seems to have complexity beyond our power of total comprehension; and medicine is trying to understand and control it.

Should the Patient be Told the Truth?

Medical practitioners continually debate whether patients should be told the "truth" about their health conditions. Like all science, medicine is based on probability. A physician may be able to predict that the chances are 99 out of 100 that a given patient will experience certain specific physiological outcomes. But even here the imprecision of science is evident. The physician cannot say with certainty that the patient will be the one case that is the exception to the prediction. Furthermore, because human conditions are not static, change is possible. Thus, today's truth may become tomorrow's lie.

Communicating truth to patients and their families is fraught with other problems. People attach different meanings to words. This is especially true of words associated with sickness. For example, "cancer" and "heart attack" have negative connotations to most lay persons. Using the best words is an art that few persons of any profession have mastered. Yet it is clear that the patient and his/her family have the right to know something about the illness. The question is: *What* do they have the right to know? Neil Fiore, a cancer patient, suggests that physicians give patients all the information they need but not without first understanding how each patient may interpret the information: "To many, 'cancer' means terminal illness and a protracted, painful death, with no hope of escaping either the disease or the treatment. Specific, concrete descriptions of the condition (i.e., its stage and the treatments available) are less likely to be misunderstood or to leave patients to their fantasies about what the doctor really means. This approach is especially important in treatment of children. Seemingly straightforward medical procedures such as a 'bone-marrow test' and 'dye injection' have been interpreted by frightened children as 'bow-and-arrow test' and 'die injection.'"[25]

Jean Comaroff's study of general practitioners in South Wales provides a glimpse at a general rule physicians sometimes adopt for giving information to patients: "Patients who ask about their symptoms or treatment are given simple explanations. A corollary to this is that those who ask no questions receive little information."[26] This strategy of communication reflects the power dynamics in doctor-patient interactions. A further elaboration of this strategy is that physicians tend to provide more information to patients whom they believe to be highly intelligent or socially powerful.

Some patients are reluctant to discuss their illness. This is frequently true of individuals who are scheduled for surgery. It is important that they be given information about routine hospital procedures. Most patients want to be told they will be well after their operation, but the surgeon must be careful not to set their expectations too high. J. H. Coverdale wrote, "Any explanations should be limited only by the capacity of the patients and relatives to grasp the complexities of human illness, and by the necessity of withholding information which, by alarming the patient would do more to impede than to facilitate his return to health."[27]

Patients with particular problems, i.e. those who have suffered a myocardial infarction and those who have undergone mastectomy, colostomy, ileostomy, and hysterectomy operations should be given detailed information about x-ray procedures, suturing, electrocardiography, and radiotherapy. Verbal and written communication should complement each other because both are indispensible components in educating patients. There is a difference between "education" and "information." Almost all patients receive information of some kind but few of them understand it and utilize it correctly. Patient education is a process of understanding medical information and complying with the health plan. Compliance should never be assumed; every patient is potentially noncompliant. The goal of physician communication with patients is to provide them with information they are able to understand and utilize.

Dying and Death

Perhaps the most difficult medical topics to deal with are dying and death. Most patients and medical practitioners fight the thought of death. Some physicians believe that they must save every patient—even those labeled "terminal." Mumford and Skipper wrote, "Without being aware of how much they demand of themselves, such persons can experience a disturbing sense of personal discomfort when they face the dying patient. Death is a

painful reminder of the realistic limits of the science of medicine
and the skills of the medical professional, as well as a reminder of
human mortality."[28]

A dying patient left this poem for medical personnel to read
after her death:

> I huddle warm inside my corner bed,
> Watching the other patients sipping tea.
> I wonder why I'm so long getting well,
> And why it is no one will talk to me.
>
> The nurses are so kind. They brush my hair
> On days I feel too ill to read or sew.
> I smile and chat, try not to show my fear,
> They cannot tell me what I want to know.
>
> The visitors come in. I see their eyes
> Become embarrassed as they pass my bed.
> "What lovely flowers!" they say, then hurry on,
> In case their faces show what can't be said.
>
> The chaplain passes on his weekly round
> With friendly smile and calm, untroubled brow.
> He speaks with deep sincerity of life,
> I'd like to speak of death, but don't know how.
>
> The surgeon comes, with student retinue,
> Mutters to sister, deaf to my pleas.
> I want to tell this dread I feel inside,
> But they are all too kind to talk to me.
>
> —*Anonymous*

As a whole, physicians pay little attention to dying patients.
They spend less time with terminally ill patients and, when
visiting them, seem to have even less to say. Medical science has
provided little room in its activities for dying or the natural and
inevitable process of death. Physicians are much more at ease
postponing death or relieving physical pain than treating a dying
person in psychological pain. Individuals whose major concerns
are therapy and cure have great difficulty discussing death with
patients.

Yet, in their more lucid moments, most physicians acknowledge that death is not a tragedy for persons such as the man whose
stroke leaves him with a live body but a dead brain. His relatives

feel grief and relief when he is finally pronounced dead and all
life support systems removed. Bereavement may contribute to the
development of physical illnesses. Grief is a universal human
phenonmenon, but few physicians seem to grasp the essential
psychological verities of the experience. Poets come closer than
most persons to capturing its essence.

> Grief fills the room of my absent child,
> Lies in his bed, walks up and down with me,
> Puts on his pretty looks, repeats his words,
> Remembers me of all his gracious parts,
> Stuffs out his vacant garments with his form.
> —*Shakespeare, King John,* act iii, scene 4

The grieving person typically tries to refute, to deny, and to
dispute the reality of the loss. It is not easy to accept the loss of
individuals taken for granted. While not a rigid order of events,
grieving tends to follow this sequence: (1) shock and disbelief, (2)
conscious awareness of the death and its meaning, (3) mourning,
and (4) resolution. Some individuals never reach the last stage.
Until physicians receive adequate coursework and clinical experiences focusing on dying patients, dying and death will be poorly
handled.

Recent studies suggest that most people, both the sick and the
well, want to know their medical diagnosis and would feel helped
more than harmed by news of terminal illnesses.[29,30] A 1977 study
of 264 physicians concluded that 98 percent of the respondents
supported being totally frank with patients who have cancer, and
all respondents said they would want to be told if they had
cancer.[31]

As noted earlier, physicians should use statistics with great
care. It is impossible to make a knowledgeable prediction about a
patient's chances of recovering without knowing how he/she
compares with the norm and also what are his/her physical and
psychological resources. In blunt terms, a physician does not
know exactly how long a specific patient will live. Nothing is
gained and much may be lost by announcing borderline findings
to a patient. Imagine the confusion aroused, Henry D. Lederer
cautions, by informing a patient, "I don't think you have much to
worry about. Your heart seems O.K., but we want to watch your
electrocardiogram because it was a little abnormal."[32]

The historical record indicates physicians have recognized that words can wound as deeply as knives, that what is said can be as significant as what is done. Those who argue that disclosure of threatening news should be the rule rather than the exception bear weighty burdens. They must have prepared themselves to learn spoken and silent cues patients telegraph about facts they know or crave about their illnesses, to communicate effectively with patients and sustain them emotionally once the news is out, to understand psychological difficulties that can accompany disclosure, and to allocate time for the often lengthy period over which disclosure can take place. They must also recognize that the harm created by inadequate mastery of the techniques and skills of communicating bad news may outweigh the benefits to the individual of learning the truth.[33]

Only by coming to terms with the feelings that the dying patient arouses in them will physicians be optimally responsive to patient needs. Inability to do so may result in a physician incorrectly telling a patient that she "will recover" or "be all right." On the other hand, it is important to note that the dying patient should not be treated like all other patients. There are many unfinished business items that most dying patients and their families would like to complete.

If the patient is a member of an identifiable family unit, it is essential for the physician to incorporate the family into the care process. Frequently physicians provide family members with the least important (from the family's perspective) information. Relatives of critically ill patients in Nancy C. Molter's study stated that they preferred (1) to know the prognosis, (2) to have their questions answered honestly, (3) to know specific facts concerning the patient's progress, (4) to receive information about the patient once a day, and (5) to have explanations given in terms that are understandable. The least helpful but most frequent messages received (1) talked about negative feelings, such as guilt or anger, (2) encouraged them to cry, (3) told about someone to help with family problems, and (4) told about other people who could help with problems.[34]

Patricia H. Butcher described the special needs of relatives of patients with brain death. Succinctly, these needs are (1) to be gently told about the illness in order to avoid false hope and (2) to be introduced to other professionals who may be able to offer spiritual and concrete support.[35] Clearly, these needs differ from those outlined by Molter. This serves to dramatize the need to know what is helpful to both patients and their relatives.

All persons in pain or who have lost a part of their body or kin have the right to grieve. Somehow the physician must be able to communicate to patients that it is all right to grieve. A more controversial issue is the physician's right to grieve. It is erroneous to assume that physicians must be superhuman persons insensitive to human suffering. However, the appropriate place for physician grieving seems to be away from patients and their families.

THE HATEFUL PATIENT

There is yet another human relations issue that we will discuss—problem patients. Because of the way they look, smell, talk or behave, some patients frustrate or irritate physicians. Patients who do not fit constantly shifting and highly subjective normative characteristics of "good" patients are labeled "problems," "undesirable," and "hateful."

Solomon Papper placed undesirable patients in five categories: socially undesirable, attitudinally undesirable, physically undesirable, circumstantially undesirable, and incidentally undesirable.[36] The socially undesirable patient includes individuals who are poverty-stricken, aged, alcoholic, members of ethnic minority groups, dirty and uneducated, and other culturally different persons. Attitudinally undesirable patients are individuals who are ungrateful, "want to know too much," "think they know so much," and those who "know a great deal." Physically undesirable patients include individuals who do not have an identifiable physical illness as well as those who have physical illnesses, especially chronic illnesses. Sometimes patients are undesirable because of circumstances totally apart from them and beyond their control. Examples of circumstantially undesirable patients are individuals who arrive at the end of a busy day and patients visiting understaffed, overcrowded, inadequately equipped clinics. Finally, the research interest of the physician may cause him/her to be less enthusiastic treating patients who do not have the illnesses characterizing his/her research.

James E. Groves focused on specific patient behavior that can earn them the "hateful patient" label. He lists four classes of such patients: dependent clingers, entitled demanders, manipulative help-rejectors, and self-destructive deniers.

> Clingers escalate from mild and appropriate requests for reassurance to repeated perfervid, incarcerating cries for explanation, affection, analgesics, sedatives and all forms of attention imaginative . . . . Demanders resemble clingers in the profundity of their neediness, but they differ in that—rather than flattery and unconscious seduction—they use intimidation, devaluation and guilt-induction to place the doctor in the role of the inexhaustible supply depot. . . . Help-rejectors, or "crocks," are familiar to every practicing physician. Like clingers and demanders, they appear to have a quenchless need for emotional supplies. Unlike clingers, they are not seductive and grateful; unlike demanders, they are not overtly hostile. They actually seem the opposite of entitled; they appear to feel that no regimen will help. . . . Self-destructive deniers display unconsciously self-murderous behaviors, such as continued drinking of a patient with esophageal varices and hepatic failure.[37]

Most clinical instructors admonish medical students to treat all patients fairly and skillfully. In short, they are told that as professionals they do not have to like patients in order to help them. It does little good to tell someone that he has a negative attitude and should change it. First, he must understand the attitude. Second, he must believe that it is counter to his professional or moral code of conduct. Finally, he must want to change. Sometimes this means undoing a lifetime of prejudice.

CULTURAL AND EDUCATIONAL CONDITIONING

Physicians' behavior is the outgrowth of ways their significant other persons—in and outside the medical profession—interpret and cope with their environment and the people in it. Prejudices based on racist and sexist beliefs and behaviors are difficult but not impossible to abate.

Cultural Diversity

America is a nation of great cultural diversity. Although all segments of our population share certain common elements of life patterns and basic beliefs, there are significant differences in subcultural attitudes, interests, goals, and dialects. Physicians bring to medical settings different cultural perceptions of masculine and feminine roles, as well as preference for certain ethnic groups and social classes.

It is well documented that racism and sexism are prevalent in the health care industry. The number and type of jobs plus the low quality of patient care available to ethnic minorities and women attest to the slowness of these conditions to change. Traditionally, health related education and employment for Third World people and women have been greatly restricted. Even with opportunities increasing due to concerted civil rights efforts at the federal and state levels, the absolute numbers of Third World people and women in the medical schools and health related professions is small compared to the proportion of the total population they represent.

Masculine and feminine roles

Until recently, in our culture, males and females were expected to play different roles. One of the first lessons children learned from adults around them was that their behavior must accord with that generally considered appropriate to their sex. A boy was not expected to take on feminine characteristics; a girl was handicapped if she was not feminine in dress, speech and aspirations. "Good boys" and "good girls" were those who engaged in sex-appropriate behavior. Gradually, sex stereotyping is disappearing—even in medicine. But the treatment still accorded women patients often is cruel and unhelpful.

> It is a mystery why physicians are so willing to cut, drug, and bully women. But they do. A hundred years ago, surgery was often performed with the explicit goal of "taming" a high-strung woman. Clitoridectomy and ovariotomy were the methods of preference then. Now, similar results are obtained by telling women that their illnesses are of psychologic origins and then treating them with tranquilizers, psychiatric therapy, shock, or institutionalization. Hysterectomies appear to be another favorite treatment and there is growing concern that many or most hysterectomies may be performed without proper indications. The surgeons' preference for radical mastectomies, in the presence of clear evidence of their emotional trauma and equally unclear evidence of their curative superiority, is also disturbing. Yet, while this cutting and drugging is going on, pelvic examinations are not performed routinely, and many physicians do not teach women patients breast examination.[38]

Most medical school lecturers use the male pronoun "he" to refer to hypothetical patients, except when discussing a patient with a disease of psychogenic origin. In the latter instance, the lecturer tends to use the female pronoun "she." Generally, females are characterized as having uninteresting illnesses, being unreliable historians, and displaying emotional rather than physical illnesses. A review of recent gynecology and urology textbooks would lead an uninformed reader to believe the physiology of micturition in females is either not well understood or not important enough to discuss. The statistically significant differences between male and female pelvic anatomy and physiology are given little attention in medical schools. Mary C. Howell wrote: "Coupled with the slights to female patients in medical-school teaching of information and skills are the attitudes and assumptions about 'woman's place' that color the doctor-patient relation. Mothers are 'complaining,' young women are 'cute tricks,' and age-peers are 'demanding and bitchy.' To quote . . . from a student: One lecturer said, 'The only significant difference between a woman and a cow is that the cow has more spigots.'"[39]

As more women patients become sensitive to physician-patient communication, there is an increasing resentment to being called "dear," "honey," and "girl" by male physicians. Male physicians using these words run the risk of being viewed as patronizing and condescending persons.

Ethnic groups

Nearly every American can trace his/her ancestry back to some country across the seas. Each ethnic group has enriched our culture with its own particular type of music, food, customs, and dress. It usually takes two or more generations for the members of a new ethnic group to become sufficiently absorbed into the life of the community so that they lose their separate identity. Some ethnic groups—mainly those of the Third World—never achieve assimilation. The assimilation of the more recent immigrant groups seems to be problematical: most of them are of the lower socioeconomic classes, and they tend to maintain their traditional beliefs, attitudes, and behavior.

Ethnic groups are generally identified by distinctive patterns of family life, language, and customs that set them apart from other groups. Above all else, members of ethnic groups feel a sense of identity and common fate. While ethnicity is frequently used to

mean race, it extends beyond race. Many ethnic minority
individuals do not use "standard" English as their first language.
The language of a people captures the essence of their culture.

Spanish, black English, and eastern and southern dialects are
examples of languages and speech patterns that not only serve as
effective barriers to patient communication but may also interfere
with the patients' ability to understand physicians. Black English
illustrates this point. Physicians who do not understand African-
American dialect may not correctly interpret the messages of
patients speaking it.

> There is increasing evidence that the differences of Afro speech from
> Anglo speech are mainly due to the survival of characteristics of African
> languages among black people in America. For instance, the *th* sound
> is absent in many West African languages, so many Afros substitute *d* as
> in *de book* or *dis* or *dat*. . . . Another example of some of the differences
> between Afro dialect and standard English dialect is the tendency to
> drop final consonants, like *ed*, *s*, or *t*. So you might hear *tes* for *test* or
> *col* for *cold*. In some cases, the final *th* becomes *f* or *t*, as in *oaf* for *oath*
> or *bof* for *both*. The *r* in *store* or *door* might be left out, so you hear *sto*
> or *do*.
>
> Afro dialect finds uses for double and multiple negatives, usually for
> emphasis: "You ain't gone find me at no touchie-feelie sensitivity
> session at no time soon!" Still another interesting characteristic of Afro
> dialect has no counterpart in "standard" English: The use of the verb *to
> be* in a continuous present tense. Thus, "she be scheming" means she
> schemed in the past, is probably scheming now, and will most likely be
> scheming in the future.[40]

Culturally enlightened physicians know that a non-Anglo or
nonstandard English language is neither better nor worse than
Anglo language; it is merely different.

Doctors who do not know the various social class dimensions
of ethnic minorities also are unlikely to know that despite
common language, color, and historical backgrounds, all members of a particular minority group are not alike. It is presump-
tuous and counterproductive to talk about *the* blacks or *the*
Indians or *the* Latins as if members of these and other groups only
have one set of behavior characteristics. While this text will focus
on general patient characteristics, the reader is reminded that
social class differences are often more determinant of a patient's
behavior than ethnic background. Third World individuals from
middle-class oriented families tend to be much more ready to fit
medical routines.

Medical School Conditioning

Some thought should be given to physicians who ostensibly have everything in their favor when working with patients from their own sex or ethnic group. There are several factors that frequently mitigate against them being optimally effective. First and foremost, most female and nonwhite physicians are Anglo-Saxon in terms of their training and professional associations. They are, in short, carbon copies of their white male colleagues. Of course, some female and nonwhite physicians are able to maintain their sexual and/or ethnic identities with a minimum loss in credibility. In terms of their verbal and nonverbal communication, however, many female and nonwhite physicians appear condescending to women and Third World patients.

In other instances, female and nonwhite physicians may feel quite marginal—estranged from white males and no longer comfortable with members of their own sexual or ethnic group. These physicians appear cold and detached to male and female, white and nonwhite patients. Another problem is the possibility that female and Third World patients will displace to women and Third World physicians their hostility toward white males.

A related issue seldom explored in depth is the lack of empathy and sensitivity physicians have for patients other than their own ethnic group. Indians, for example, display considerable hostility toward blacks, and Mexican-Amercians frequently reject Chinese-Americans. No doubt you can think of other illustrations. It is worth noting at this juncture that all Americans are products of institutionalized racism and sexism, and awareness of this fact will allow each physician to better deal with his/her own racism or sexism.

Caucasian male physicians—who constitute the overwhelming majority of members in medical associations—are beginning to come to grips with their own sexism and racism and that of their colleagues. Ideally, such introspection will not lead to a repression or denial of hostile feelings. Nor should a physician who is trying to understand his/her sexism and racism be immobilized by guilt. *Proactive* rather than inactive physicians are needed if the vicious circles of racism and sexism are to be broken.

In the end, ethnic and sex similarities are not adequate

substitutes for physicians who are (1) linguistically compatible with patients, (2) empathic, and (3) well trained. This means that the initial edge minority group or female physicians may have with female or minority group patients will be lost if these doctors cannot get beyond their ethnic history and sexual identity.

THE READINGS

The readings that follow present explicit and implicit statements about the role of communication in patient care. Some of the communication skills needed for effective patient care include being a good listener, recognizing the patient's as well as one's own self-interests and needs, being empathic and flexible, having a sense of timing, utilizing the patient's resources, and giving relevant information.

An effective physician listens in a way that he/she is really able to hear what the patient is trying to say. This does not mean telling the patient what to say. Being empathic means identifying with the other person's point of view. Meaningful communication is impossible without empathy. An effective physician understands himself/herself and tries to gain similar understanding of the patient. Self-knowledge is a prerequisite to helping others. In the quest for self-knowledge, it is important to be flexible. Rarely is there one answer or a single interpretation for an event or situation. Furthermore, there will be instances in which patients may ask physicians to give them answers when they really need help in finding their own answers.

Unless physicians understand diverse cultural norms and values, they may intervene at the wrong time or with the wrong family members. Above all else, the physician must help the patient to effectively use scientific knowledge, techniques, and medicine. This is best done with language that the patient understands. Help is only help when it is perceived as such. Little good is likely to be accomplished if a physician uses unexplained jargon or belittles folk cultures.

While the readings that follow are exemplary of methods and techniques for improving physician-patient communication, they are not exhaustive. You should read other materials and carefully devise humane methods and techniques of communication that fit your own personality and work situation.

REFERENCES

1. Roger J. Bulger (Ed.), *Hippocrates Revisited: A Search for Meaning*. New York: Medcom, 1973, p. 66.
2. David E. Reiser, Struggling to stay human in medicine: one student's reflections on becoming a doctor. *New Physician, 22*:297,1973.
3. *Ibid.*, p. 298.
4. Prakash Burra and Alexander M. Bryans, The helping professions group: interpersonal dimensions in health sciences education. *J Med Educ, 54*:39, 1979.
5. David K. Berlo, *The Process of Communication: An Introduction to Theory and Practice*. New York: Holt, Rinehart & Winston, 1960, p. 24.
6. Donald W. Johnson, *Reaching Out: Interpersonal Effectiveness and Self-Actualization*. Englewood Cliffs, NJ: Prentice-Hall, 1972, p. 62.
7. Harold D. Lasswell, The structure and function of communication in society. In L. Bryson (Ed.), *The Communication of Ideas*. New York: Harper & Row, 1948, p. 37.
8. Dean C. Barnlund, Toward a meaning-centered philosophy of communication. *J Communications, 11*:198-292, 1962.
9. Jurgen Ruesch and Gregory Bateson, *Communication: The Social Matrix of Psychiatry*. New York: W. W. Norton, 1951, pp. 5-6.
10. Claude Shannon and Warren Weaver, *The Mathematical Theory of Communication*. Urbana: University of Illinois Press, 1949.
11. W. L. Schramm, *The Processes and Effects of Mass Communications*. Urbana: University of Illinois Press, 1954.
12. Berlo, *loc.cit.*
13. Emily Mumford and James K. Skipper, Jr., *Sociology in Hospital Care*. New York: Harper & Row, 1967, p. 123.
14. How nurses rate hospital care. *Time*, January 15, 1977, p. 3.
15. Patients err on machine, study finds. *Raleigh [NC] News and Observer*, January 13, 1977.
16. Daniel M. Laskin, The doctor-patient relationship: a potential communication gap. *J Oral Surgery, 37*:786, 1979.
17. Harry E. Munn, Jr., Communication between patients, nurses, physicians and surgeons, *Hosp Topics, 55*:7, 1977.
18. Edward T. Hall, *The Silent Language*. New York: Doubleday, 1959.
19. Mumford and Skipper, Jr., *op.cit.*, p. 125.
20. D. J. G. Bain, Doctor-patient communication in general practice consultations. *J Med Educ, 10*:125, 1976.
21. P. S. Bryne and B. E. L. Long, *Doctors Talking to Patients*. London: Department of Health and Social Security, 1976.
22. D. J. G. Bain, The content of physician-patient communication in family practice. *J. Fam Pract, 8*:745-53, 1979.
23. Bain, *loc.cit.*
24. G. R. Foster, Jr., The magic word in the effective practice of medicine. *J Medical Assn Georgia, 68*:708, 1979.
25. Neil Fiore, Fighting cancer—one patient's perspective. *New Engl J Med, 300*:287, 1979.

26. Jean Comaroff, Communicating information about non-fatal illness: the strategies of a group of general practitioners. *Sociological Rev, 27:*274, 1976.

27. J. H. Coverdale, Doctor-patient communication: the example of communicating with the peptic ulcer patient. *New Zealand Med J, 89:*221-2, 1979.

28. Mumford and Skipper, *op.cit.,* p. 203.

29. S. Bok, *Lying: Moral Choice in Public and Private Life.* New York: Pantheon Books, 1978, p. 229.

30. M. Blumenfied, N. B. Levy, and D. Kaufman, Do patients want to be told the truth? *MGH News, 38:*7-8, 1979.

31. D. H. Novack, E. J. Freireich, and S. Vaisrub, Changes in physician attitudes toward telling the cancer patient. *JAMA, 241:*897-900, 1979.

32. Henry D. Lederer, How the sick view their world. *J Soc Issues, 8:*159, 1952.

33. Stanley J. Reiser, Words as scalpels: transmitting evidence in the clinical dialogue. *Ann Intern Med, 92:*840-1, 1980.

34. Nancy C. Molter, Needs of relatives of critically ill patients: a descriptive study. *Heart Lung, 8:*334, 1979.

35. Patricia H. Butcher, Management of relatives of patients with brain death. *Anesthesiology Clin, 17:*327-32, 1979.

36. Solomon Papper, The undesirable patient. *J Chron Dis, 22:*771-9, 1970.

37. James E. Groves, Taking care of the hateful patient. *New Engl J Med, 291:*305, 1974.

38. Jerry L. Weaver and Sharon D. Garrett, Sexism and racism in the American health care industry: a comparative analysis. *Internat J Health Serv, 8:*695, 1978.

39. Marcy C. Howell, What medical schools teach about women. *New Engl J Med, 291:*305, 1974.

40. Clyde Taylor, Soul talk: a key to black cultural attitudes. In Dorothy Luckraft (Ed.), *Black Awareness: Implications for Black Patient Care,* New York: American Journal of Nursing, 1976, pp. 1-2.

Chapter 2

DOCTOR-PATIENT COMMUNICATION

BARBARA M. KORSCH AND VIDA FRANCIS NEGRETE

The problem of dissatisfaction with the delivery of medical care in the U.S. is not solely a matter of inadequate financing or insufficient facilities and personnel. When all is said and done, it remains obvious that improvement of the funding and availability of medical service, although essential, would not in itself be a sufficient answer to the problem. The quality of medical care depends in the last analysis on the interaction of the patient and the doctor, and there is abundant evidence that in current practice this interaction all too often is disappointing to both parties. Systematic surveys confirm that there is widespread dissatisfaction among patients with doctors and among doctors with lack of cooperation by their patients.

Of the various factors that tend to contribute to this discontent, certainly one of the most important is poor communication between doctor and patient. In modern medical practice, which is now focused predominantly on technical knowledge, the physician may be engrossed in technical concerns and arcane terminology that mystify the patient. The traditional system of a close, long-term relationship with a "family doctor" is being replaced for the patient by short-term encounters with specialists. Moreover, many physicians no longer attach high importance to personal rapport with the patient; to some the "bedside manner" seems a concession to salesmanship not befitting a medical scientist. As we shall see, however, the failure to establish empathy with patients can be a serious bar to communication

Reprinted with permission from *Scientific American,* 227:66-74. Copyright © 1972 by Scientific American, Inc. All rights reserved.

and patient response. (Indeed, the common neglect of this
psychological factor by doctors may account in part for the
flourishing of quacks and faith healers, whose main attraction
for sick people is their skill in furnishing emotional reassurance.)

As an illustration of the critical importance of the personal
interaction of patient and doctor, let us consider a not untypical
case. A mother in a state of high anxiety about the persistent
severe coughing of her infant son takes him to a hospital clinic.
The physician, without greeting her or addressing her by name,
asks a few matter-of-fact questions and examines the baby. He
finds that the child has a postnasal drip of mucus (from an
inflamed sinus) that is causing the cough. Without explaining
the cause to the mother, the doctor simply prescribes nose drops,
steam inhalation and perhaps an antibiotic and asks the mother
to return with the baby in a couple of days for a follow-up
examination. The mother, disappointed that the doctor has
apparently shown no concern about her distress over the baby's
cough, and unable to see how the prescriptions could stop or
relieve the cough, buys cough medicine at the corner drugstore
instead of using the prescribed treatment. She does not go back to
the doctor for a follow-up. If the cough actually betokened a
serious underlying condition, she has left the baby in jeopardy.
The physician, for his part, writes her off as an uncooperative
parent because she has not returned.

Over the past five years our research team at the Childrens
Hospital of Los Angeles, associated with the University of
Southern California School of Medicine, has been investigating
the important problem of doctor-patient communication. Obviously this is a crucial but neglected aspect of medical care.
Medical schools do an admirable job of teaching their students
the complexities of medical science, but they still leave the
learning of the "art" of medical practice to the individual's own
initiative and intuition. This remains, in our view, a serious
omission. However well informed a physician may be, and
however conscientious about applying his knowledge, if he
cannot get his message across to the patient, his competence is not
going to be helpful. Moreover, more than half of a physician's
working time in patient care, particularly in fields such as
general practice, pediatrics and internal medicine, is spent on

problems involving primarily psychological factors and the need for communication rather than technical knowledge. Consequently, detailed study of the process of communication between doctors (or other health professionals) and patients is essential for improvement of the delivery of medical care. By clarifying the process we can hope to develop principles that will make it possible to teach something about the "art of medicine" in medical school, instead of leaving it solely to intuition.

There have been many studies of factors influencing the response of patients to medical counsel and treatment: factors such as the patient's background, personality and previous medical contacts, and on the other hand, the doctor's personal characteristics and training. For our study we had to find a setting and a technique that would enable us to examine selectively the doctor-patient communication process itself. How could we arrange to isolate this factor? We chose a simple but natural situation that seemed to answer our needs. The patient sample would be a large one, representing a mixed population of diverse ethnic, social, economic and cultural backgrounds. Similarly, the doctor sample visited by these patients would also be sizable. In each instance the patient would visit a physician the patient had not met before and would present a case of acute illness (not previously diagnosed or treated) for which the physician could prescribe some definite treatment or course of action by the patient. The entire interview would be recorded, and afterward a member of our research team would follow up to learn how the patient responded to the interview and the doctor's instructions.

The situation we sought was well fulfilled by the emergency clinic of the Childrens Hospital. Children are brought to this walk-in clinic with a great variety of acute (but seldom catastrophic) illnesses or accidental injuries, invariably accompanied by a parent. The visit is usually short and generally yields a specific recommendation from the doctor to the parent. The clinic has a large staff of pediatricians, mostly young, well-trained, full-time residents. In our basic study we observed 800 visits by 800 different patients. Since the interaction was mainly between the child's mother and the doctor, we designated the mother as the "patient." Our standard procedure was to make an audio tape recording of the entire interview, then question the mother immediately afterward concerning what she had expected from the visit and what her reactions to it were and finally follow up later (within 14 days) to learn whether or not she had complied with the physician's instructions.

The setting and procedure provided a number of controls that minimized complication of the findings by extraneous factors, that is, variables other than the ones we wished to investigate. Since the patient came to a new physician to consider an acute illness not yet diagnosed or treated, the doctor-patient communication about the situation consisted only of the interchange between the two parties during this visit, uncomplicated by previous transactions or by any prior briefing of the parent about the illness. The large size of the samples (both of patients and of physicians) tended to correct for the bias of extraneous personal factors such as social or educational background when the responses of the group as a whole were considered. (Actually we found on analyzing the results that most patients, regardless of their personal background, responded to a given communication style in much the same way.) Another factor we had to consider was the possibility that the tape-recording of the visit might cause the doctor to depart from his usual style and put his best foot forward, so to speak. It turned out, however, that in most cases the physician disregarded the presence of the tape recorder and behaved naturally. As a control, we omitted the use of the tape recorder in 300 of the 800 visits, and we found this apparently made no difference in the physicians' performance or the patients' reactions to the interview.

The findings from the 800 cases have since been supplemented with hundreds of other observations of doctor-patient communication, many of them involving routine checkups of well children, many not in clinics but in the private practice of pediatricians. In general these observations confirmed the validity of the conclusions from the basic study. It must still be borne in mind that the setting for that study was after all rather special: an emergency visit in a clinic on an acute but usually minor illness, generally with a young doctor of only brief pediatric experience (one to three years). The patient's response in a case of severe chronic illness or to a physician of long acquaintance might well have been very different. Our concern, however, was to look into the effects of particular modes of communication (or noncommunication) irrespective of other factors. The barriers to communication that were spotlighted in our study may occur in any setting, although they are not as common or as severe in private practice as they are in a single emergency visit to a clinic.

What, then, were the findings in detailed analysis of the 800 clinic visits? We consider first the mothers' evaluation of the conference with the physician. Immediately after the visit a member of our research team interviewed each parent to ascertain how she had felt about the child's illness, what she had expected of the doctor and how well satisfied she was with what he had said and done. Of the entire group, 40 percent were highly satisfied, 36 percent moderately satisfied, 11 percent moderately dissatisfied and 13 percent highly dissatisfied. That 76 percent of these anxious mothers were more or less satisfied with the doctor's performance in their brief encounter in the clinic is of course a reassuring finding. Their specific reactions, however, were less favorable. Nearly a fifth (149) of the 800 mothers felt they had not received a clear statement of what was wrong with their baby, and almost half of the entire group were still wondering when they left the physician what had caused their child's illness. The absence of an explanation of the cause is unnerving in such a situation, because the mother of a sick baby generally has a tendency to blame herself for the occurrence and needs specific reassurance.

The subsequent follow-up on how the mothers complied with the physician's instructions told a disquieting story. We took pains to obtain a true account by asking the mother searching but tactful questions (such as "When were you able to discontinue the treatment?") and by checking medicine bottles or the pharmacy when feasible. It turned out that 42 percent of the mothers had carried out all of the doctor's medical advice, 38 percent had complied only in part and 11 percent not at all. (In the remaining 8 percent of the cases the physician had not felt it necessary to give any prescription or advice.)

As was to be expected, we found a substantial correlation between the mothers' expressed satisfaction with the doctor's behavior in the visit and their compliance with his instruction. Of the highly satisfied mothers 53.4 percent cooperated completely with his advice, whereas only 16.7 percent of the highly dissatisfied patients did so. The fact that the correlation between compliance and satisfaction with the doctor was not consistenly observed can be attributed to complicating factors such as the mothers' view of the seriousness of the illness, the complexity of the physician's instruction, the difficulty of the prescribed treatment and various practical problems.

For light on the specific problems of communication between doctor and patient we now turn to detailed analysis of the content of their interchanges as recorded verbatim in the tapes. We coded the various features or elements characterizing their conversations and the patients' reactions and then submitted the data to analysis by computer. One of the tools we used was an adaptation of the "interaction process analysis" technique of the psychologist Robert F. Bales, which describes the content and tone of verbal interaction in terms of affect—positive and negative.

A question that immediately comes to mind with regard to a doctor-patient interview is the influence of the length of the session. It is commonly supposed that the more time the doctor can spend with the patient, the more satisfactory the results will be. No doubt part of the dissatisfaction with present medical care is attributable to the limited time harried physicians can give their patients. Surprisingly, however, the results of our study indicated that time was not necessarily of the essence. The 800 visits we examined varied in length from two minutes to 45 minutes, and we could find no significant correlation between the length of the session and (1) the patient's satisfaction or (2) the clarity of the diagnosis of the child's illness. Indeed, on examining some of the longest sessions we noted that the time was consumed largely by failures in communication: the doctor and patient were spending the time trying to get on the same wavelength!

The general impression that physicians tend to be too technical in language for their patients is strongly confirmed by our study. Terms such as nares, peristalsis and Coombs titre were Greek to the patients. A "lumbar puncture" was interpreted as meaning an operation to drain the lungs, and a reference to "incubation period" was taken to signify the length of time the sick child was to be kept in bed. A mother who was told that her child would be "admitted for a work-up" did not realize that he was to be hospitalized; when another mother was told by the physician that he would have to "explore," she had no idea he was talking about surgery. In more than half of the cases we recorded the physicians resorted to medical jargon. This did not necessarily leave the patient dissatisfied; some patients were impressed and even flattered by such language. It did, however, leave most of the mothers unenlightened about the nature of the child's illness. One of the interesting findings was that satisfaction with the doctor's communication was not significantly higher among college-educated mothers than it was among those with less education.

The language barrier was by no means the most serious bar to effective communication. The severest and most common complaint of the dissatisfied mothers was that the physician had shown too little interest in their great concern about their child. High among the expectations of mothers in coming to the clinic was that the doctor would be friendly and sympathetic not only to the child but also to the worried parent. The recordings show, however, that less than 5 percent of the physician's conversation was personal or friendly in nature. In most of the visits the physician gave no attention to the mother's own feelings and devoted himself solely to technical discussion of the child's condition. The disregard of the mother's concern must be considered an important hindrance to communication in the light of the fact that, as we found in the postvisit interviews, 300 of the 800 mothers held themselves in some way responsible for their child's illness. In a few instances the physician even expressly blamed, or appeared to blame, the mother. In one case a physician remarked to the child, perhaps in jest, "Stevie, it's your mother's fault that you have this high fever." The mother later voiced great distress over this to our interviewer.

A frequent cause of dismay for the mother was the physician's total disregard of her account of what chiefly worried her about the child's illness. When, for instance, a mother repeatedly tried to interest the doctor in the fact that her child had been vomiting, he ignored her remarks and persisted in asking her about other symptoms, which, as she did not realize, related to the same basic problem—dehydration of the child. Another mother feared that her child's febrile convulsions might cause permanent damage to the brain, but she did not succeed in engaging the doctor's attention to this concern. Among the 800 mothers, 26 percent told interviewers after the session with the doctor that they had not mentioned their greatest concern to the physician because they did not have an opportunity or were not encouraged to do so.

Under such circumstances there was frequently a complete breakdown of communication. Some patients were so preoccupied with their dominant concerns that they were unable to listen to the physician. Some even reported that the physician had failed to examine the child adequately or to give a prescription, although the tape-recorded account of the visit attests that he did in fact do so. Among mothers who felt that the physician had not understood their concerns 68 percent were dissatisfied with the visit, whereas of the 625 mothers who reported the physician had understood, 83 percent were satisfied.

We have mentioned that 149 patients reported they had not been told what was the matter with their sick child. The recordings of the visits show that in many cases the physician did indeed fail to provide a clear diagnostic statement, and often he offered no prognosis. Diagnosis was of course one of the main expectations that had brought each mother to the clinic. Many of the mothers complied with the doctor's medical advice even when no diagnosis was given. Understandably, however, omission of such important information did not tend to inspire confidence in his prescriptions. Only 54 of the 800 patients seriously questioned the physician's technical competence (in their postvisit interviews with us), but failure to show a friendly interest or to fulfill their other expectations was a significant deterrent to compliance with his instruction. Of the patients who felt that the physician had not met any of their expectations, 56 percent were grossly noncompliant.

On the positive side, the recordings of the hundreds of doctor-patient conversations clearly identified specific forms of discourse that made for good communication and patient satisfaction. One of these, of course, was expression by the doctor of friendly interest in the "patient" with whom he was conducting the conversation (that is, the mother). Most of the physicians believed they had been friendly, but fewer than half of the patients had this impression, and 193 of them reported that the doctor had been strictly businesslike. Attention to the mother's worried concerns had a high correlation with success in satisfying her and obtaining her compliance with advice. This suggests that a physician can quickly establish fruitful communication with the patient by opening the conversation with questions such as: "Why did you bring Johnny to the clinic? . . . What worried you the most about him? . . . Why did that worry you?" A brief but friendly discussion of the patient's concerns, however irrelevant or irrational they may seem, can perform wonders in reassuring her and winning her cooperation. Even when the physician was not able to fulfill all the mother's expectations, a demonstration of warm concern and individualization of his advice achieved satisfying results. The patients reacted poorly to impersonal or institutional expressions such as "We don't hospitalize children with impetigo" or "We keep most cases of pneumonia under observation in the clinic." On the other hand, patient rapport and cooperation thrived on specific instructions, expressions of trust in the mother's caretaking ability and offers of continued interest such as "Call me anytime" or "We'll check Johnny again tomorrow."

Detailed study of the recordings with the aid of Bale's method of interaction process analysis brought forth a number of significant findings, some of them unexpected. The verbatim records showed that on the average the doctor did more talking than the mother, which proved to be a surprise to these physicians and probably comes as news to the medical fraternity generally. The session tended to have a more successful outcome when the patient had an active interchange with the doctor than it did when she remained passive and asked few questions. In general the patients were disappointingly reticent about asking questions or opening up lines of inquiry, in view of the anxiety and desire for more information that they expressed to interviewers afterward.

It may be significant in this connection that in some recordings the doctor-patient conversation comes to a distinct breaking point, after which no real communication takes place and one or the other participant is reduced to mechanical uh-huhs or yeses. In other cases the physician is found to fall into repeating statements several times and showing increasing impatience and irritation. These two types of situations probably reflect great tension on the part of the patient as well as the collapse of communication.

The verbal records give relatively few obvious signs of affect. Civilities between the parties, such as introducing themselves or addressing each other by name, are uncommon. The interchanges consist mainly of neutral, informational statements. Nevertheless, the tone and emotional content of the encounters is amply evidenced. One noteworthy finding is that, whereas less than 6 percent of the doctor's communication to the mother carries positive affect (in the form of friendly remarks, joking, agreement, support), 46 percent of his conversation with the child is of this nature. Plainly the physician not only identifies with the child rather than with the mother as the patient but also feels a need to give more reassurance to the child than he would to an adult. The results in this study, however, indicated that the physician's friendliness to the child had only a slight influence in heightening the mother's satisfaction with the visit or getting her to follow his medical advice. It was his attitude toward her that counted most.

If the physicians rarely show positive affect to the mother in these records, by the same token they seldom show negative affect in the form of disapproval, criticism or hostility. When the doctor does express negative feelings, the mother is likely to be dissatisfied with the visit and fail to comply with his advice. Conversely, a substantial showing of positive affect by the doctor to the mother enhances her satisfaction and compliance. This finding has a bearing on a controversial issue in medical practice. There is a widely held belief that the doctor should maintain a certain social distance from the patient to strengthen his image as a figure of authority, and some physicians go so far as to use scare techniques to obtain compliance with their advice, threatening dire consequences if it is not followed. Some patients seek out this type of doctor; they may in fact need such treatment. In our investigation, however, we came across few such individuals. Friendly treatment of the patient generally had favorable results; harsh treatment tended to yield poor results. And there was a direct statistical relation between the amount of nonmedical (that is, sociable) conversation between doctor and patient and the patient's satisfaction with the encounter with the doctor.

The patients exhibited considerably more negative affect than the physicians did. Very few of the mothers openly expressed hostility or resentment to the doctor; expressions of negative feelings usually took the form of statements indicating nervousness or tension. Such statements ran as high as 45 percent of all the utterances by the mother in some cases, and in the total sample they amounted to 10 percent of all the patients' statements. In a large number of these instances the physician did not offer any reassuring response to the mother's indication of anxiety.

Our exploration of the communication aspect of health care in some depth has opened up encouraging prospects for relatively simple ways to improve the delivery of this care. It is certainly not our intention to undermine public confidence in the medical profession; on the contrary, the lessons learned from analysis of the communication problem can go far to help the profession gain support and strengthen its performance. Whereas other problems that stand in the way of delivering health care satisfactorily to the entire population seem to call for reorganization of the entire social structure and basic personality changes in the people, the communication problem can be solved more easily.

The shortcomings in communication that we have examined in the clinic situation after all reflect a pattern that is common in medical practice generally. Furthermore, the need for understanding the problem of communication and coping with it is increasing as the delivery of medical care is taken over more and more by specialized professionals and technicians, so that the patient must relate to a galaxy of different health workers. Unquestionably attention to effective communication, a skill that should not be too difficult for any trained person to master, could make a valuable contribution to the quality of health care and its availability to the general population.

With the technique of detailed analysis that our research team has used in examining verbal communication we are looking into certain other aspects of medical practice. We have begun to make video tapes of medical visits, which enable us to study nonverbal communication and to document the "instrumental" (as distinguished from "expressive") performance of doctors, including examinations of the patient. When a body of data on all these matters, expressive and instrumental, has been developed and units of behavior in the process of health care have been clearly defined, there will be a more solid basis for establishing optimal standards and comparing actual performance with these standards. It will then be possible to measure the quality of health care, to relate the elements of the process to results in patient health and to evaluate the contribution of the social and emotional aspects of patient care. These aspects may well be found to have a far weightier influence in preserving health and well-being than they are credited with now.

Chapter 3

THE MEDICAL INTERVIEW: PROBLEMS IN COMMUNICATION

ROGER W. SHUY

P hysicians, like many other professionals, are frequently unaware of the important role which language plays in their daily encounters with patients. Although it is generally agreed, for example, that the success of treatment hinges on an accurate medical history, little or no preparation is provided in medical training for developing competence in the language and culture of the wide variety of patients which our society produces.

The factors which interfere with effective communication between patient and doctor in the medical interview can be identified. The doctor-patient encounter itself is shrouded with emotion, on the part of the patient at least. Secondly, the interview is often carried out in language which has been described by several members of the medical profession as a peculiar and technical jargon. The following is one such recent observation.

> The physician speaks a strange and often unintelligible dialect. He calls everyday common objects by absurd and antiquated terms. He speaks of mitral commissurotomies, pituitary insufficiency, and reality feedback. This world is peopled with cirrhotics, greensticks, and hebephrenics. The professional dialect creates a communication gap between physician and patient that is generally acknowledged by neither.
>
> Increased specialization refines the physician's particular dialect, and he becomes much like the computer, tolerating only the imprint of words that fit into the programmed languages.[6]

From Roger W. Shuy, The Medical Interview: Problems in Communication, *Primary Care*, 3:365-86, 1976. Reprinted with permission.

A third factor leading to interference in the effective communication between patient and doctor stems from the socioeconomic reality of our society. Medicine, as a profession, is a middle-class phenomenon. Of this, Kimball points out:

> Although medicine has traditionally been the most accessible of the professions in terms of providing for upward social mobility, it has recruited most of its manpower from the middle class, especially the upper middle class. These groups display life styles, thought processes, and a dialect far removed from those of most patients.[6]

This situation obtains equally for psychoanalysts, as Hollingsworth and Redlich clearly indicated in 1958 when they pointed out that money commands attention from psychiatrists.[4] Those who are relatively poor or uneducated are given little or no attention, and it has been estimated by one prominent psychoanalyst that an overwhelming majority of presumed successes in psychotherapy are with middle-class patients (Harley Shands, personal communication). A suitable patient, in fact, might well be defined as one who is comfortable with the language and culture of the therapist, which is, by definition, middle-class.

One obvious suggestion to overcome this middle-class bias of medicine and psychiatry is to recruit more doctors from the working classes in order to reduce this mismatch of language and culture from patient to doctor. As hopeful as this might sound, past experience has shown that there is something in the acquisition of medical knowledge which seems to wipe out former ties and culture. Casual observation of many physicians who come from the working classes has revealed a relative lack of sympathy toward patients of working-class status. Apparently the same assimilative phenomenon is at work in medicine that already has been observed in school teachers. Perhaps you can't really go home again, as Thomas Wolfe once said.

As a remedy to this mismatch of the doctor's difficulties with dialect, both with his own professional jargon and with the social and cultural dialect of the patient, Kimball suggests a refocused medical education:

> Medical schools have the opportunity to sharpen the student's hearing and to broaden his understanding of disease and illness patterns at an early and sensitive stage in his development. Unfortunately, interviewing, as a diagnostic and therapeutic skill, is ignored and underestimated by many medical faculties. Departments of medicine often

reduce interviewing to history taking. Although some emphasis is placed on past, family, and social history, the focus is directed toward disease specificity rather than the illness and its relationship to the patient, his family, and his community.[6]

Kimball suggests that one way to enlarge the medical students' experience with the dialects of the working-class community is to expose them to such groups during their training.

One medical school in the Southwest has planned a training session in clinical medicine in a neighborhood health clinic— learning interviewing techniques in the real world. In this case, the program requires that the medical students learn Spanish since most families enrolled in the neighborhood health clinic speak only that language. Obviously not much information is communicated unless the doctor learns to understand the patient in his own tongue. Not satisfied with this, Kimball further suggests: "In many of our urban medical schools physicians-in-training could use special courses in culture and language of subgroups, whether or not they speak English."[6]

In an important study of the ways in which cognitive and linguistic and conversational elements are basic to the medical history interview, Aaron V. Cicourel laments that the fixed choice questionnaire typically used by the physician obscures for analysis the reasoning processes of the interviewer. Several observations are possible nonetheless. The interview problems are treated as technical issues. Physicians give little or no credence to the possibility of training in interviewing techniques:

> The physician relies on powerful theories from biology, biochemistry and the neurosciences to justify his diagnosis and treatment; he tends to ignore the difficult interface between common sense talk to the patient, and the translation of the question-answer format into clinical science terms.

Cicourel continues:

> How stored information is organized and how access is to be made is not defined as a serious problem. The researcher assumes the respondent will be presented with "normal" speaking intonation, standardized syntactic structures, and standardized topics as indexed by the same lexical items. Open-ended questions that encourage spontaneous responses are not encouraged because this complicates the coding of responses and the achievement of a standardized format.[3]

Before such a program were to be developed, one would want to be sure that adequate knowledge existed concerning the language and culture of such subgroups. Recent research in the distinctive language patterns of Blacks, Puerto Ricans, isolated Appalachians, and minorities of other types, for example, has enlarged our potential for designating areas of communication breakdown in a number of settings. Linguistic research at Georgetown University, The University of Pennsylvania, and The Center for Applied Linguistics, for example, has pointed out the consistent, systematic linguistic contrasts between minority speech and the language of the middle-classes. Such information is useful both as a predictor of potential communication breakdown and as a critical measurement point for remediation. In the past, these linguistic descriptions have been helpful to educators in that they specify the exact nature of the problem and they enable the teacher to adhere to the long cherished (but seldom followed) notion of starting with the student where he is. That is, teaching materials can be built more efficiently after it is clearly established where the learner is on the educational continuum.

As things now stand, the typical minority group patient is in a similar position to the minority group student in the schools. Much has been said about compensatory education in recent years. In reality, what this means is that the institution (the school) does not feel that certain minority group children are culturally, socially or linguistically ready for education. To make them ready, a program is devised that will change their culture, their social behavior, and their language to conform to the expectations of the school. Compensatory education argues essentially that the child must be like the school in order for the school to be able to teach him. Current medical practice utilizes a similar communications mode. The patient must adjust to the language and culture of the physician or health professional. The medical profession does no better job of starting with its clients *where they are* than does the teaching profession. If the various medical specialists cited earlier are correct in their assessment of current practices in doctor-patient relationships, a great deal of miscommunication is taking place not simply because of the emotionally charged nature of the interaction and not simply because of the doctor's use of medical jargon, but because of a critical lack of awareness concerning the linguistic and cultural systems which some patients bring with them to the medical interview.

three: the fact that the event may be laden with patient emotion, the behavior of the doctor with respect to the language of his specialty, and the obvious class-contrast between doctor and working-class patient. All of these factors have been noted in the literature, by the medical profession as well as others. Still, relatively few hard data are available to verify or reject these assumptions. This situation results partially from the tendencies toward self-preservation by the medical profession itself, where presumed high standards of ethics have all but eliminated internal criticism. Psychiatry is probably the extreme example of this, as Brazelon[2] observes, where ". . . there are no commmonly accepted standards of good work or ways to prove that changes in a patient's life are due in fact to his clinical sessions. Success can always be imputed to the psychiatrist's impact and failure can always be attributed to the patient."[2] The National Hospital Association has been studying doctor-patient relationships and has compiled a list of the ten questions most often asked by patients. Leading the list is the question: "Why don't doctors explain a medical problem in simple language that a patient can understand?" In answer to this question, heart surgeon Michael E. DeBakey replied: "Most doctors don't want their patients to understand them! They prefer to keep their work a mystery. If patients don't understand what a doctor is talking about, they won't ask him questions. Then the doctor won't have to be bothered answering them."[8]

Recent research into the communication problems of patients has as its general purpose the extent of the miscommunication, but especially to examine how much patients feel or are led to feel that they must communicate with doctors in the doctor's own language. Conversely, we are also interested in those occasions in which doctors show a need to try to communicate with their patients in patient language. One might hypothesize a continuum such as the following:

Doctors talking only Doctor language	Doctors talking Doctor language but understanding Patient language	Doctors speaking and understanding Patient language	Patients speaking and understanding Doctor language	Patients talking Patient language but understanding Doctor language	Patients speaking only Patient language

This article addresses the following issues:

1. What evidence can be noted to determine that patients are either understanding or not understanding doctor talk?

2. What evidence can be noted to determine that doctors are either understanding or not understanding patient talk?

3. What failures and/or successes can be determined in the efforts of patients to talk doctor language?

4. What failures and/or successes can be determined in the efforts of doctors to talk patient language?

5. How can all of the above evidences, successes and failures be accounted for in terms of the known facts of language and culture?

DO PATIENTS FEEL THAT THERE IS A COMMUNICATION PROBLEM WITH THEIR DOCTORS?

Probably the most basic question we could ask in a study of such questions is whether a communication problem between doctors and patients really exists. Since our work was to be done largely at Georgetown University Hospital, it seemed useful to get at least a pilot survey of patient reactions to their care and treatment there. Effort was made to design a set of questions in the clearest possible language to avoid ambiguities and confusion. Fourteen such questions were constructed, worded and arranged so that some points would be evaluated twice (Appendix A). Five of the questions were directed at addressing the nature of the vocabulary problems between medical people and patients. Two questions attempted to assess whether or not there was something in the medical person's attitude which discouraged free communiation by the patient. Answers to questions relating to the time element and the doctor's real or apparent personal interest were sought in five questions. One question asked for the patient's overall assessment of satisfaction and one explored the possibility of undue secrecy on the part of the doctor.

The questionnaire was administered randomly to 105 patients in the waiting rooms of the various clinics and private medical practices during a two-week period at the hospital. The results demonstrate clear evidence of how widespread the problem is.

On the matter of vocabulary, 45 percent of the people (a wide age range with race and sex variation was achieved) said that they sometimes felt the doctor did not understand the patient's problem. Replying to this question with a positive answer does not relate the percentage unique to linguistic problems, of course, because other factors could be involved such as the doctor's inattention to the patient's minor or continuous complaints.

Other percentages for vocabulary problems come close to this, however; 38 percent thought that doctors, nurses, or interns sometimes use words that are difficult to understand while 45 percent thought it was sometimes difficult for the patient to explain himself to the doctor. Thirty-five percent would prefer the doctor to speak in simpler language. However, only 15 percent would say that the doctor usually *expects* you to know medical words, possibly indicating that this just happens to be the way doctors talk and that the patients are not directly blamed for not being able to understand the doctor. They would like it if the doctor could modify his language to be more easily and fully comprehended. The problem does not sit solely with the doctor as the only cause because patients admit to an equal share of the problem.

The doctor's attitude was assessed negatively by 42 percent and 51 percent of the interviewees. Thirty-nine percent felt that the doctor's attitude is sometimes unfriendly. This may stem, of course, from a large variety of causes, but the general feeling of "unfriendliness" includes most anything. Fifty-one percent felt inhibited by the doctor's attitude, personality, or style.

The inhibition seems to occur through the patient's recognition of a major difference in intellectual levels between himself and the doctor. We might infer that many patients credit the doctor with so much intelligence and preoccupation with "important matters" that they cannot bother him with minor or irrelevant questions. This is a potentially critical factor in communication because some problems, no matter how superfluous for the doctor, may be deep seated sources of worry and discomfort for the patient. If the patient holds back on these things his anxiety is not alleviated.

The medical profession is one where time seems an exceedingly valuable item. Patients see doctors as very busy people. The questionnaire reveals, though, that a sizable number of patients think that more time should be spent with them. It has been a basic assumption in our research that time is not in reality what some patients feel is lacking, but more often a larger degree of active interest and attention should be accorded them when they are with the doctor. This attention is extended through oral-linguistic means—communication. It is not so important how much time is spent with the patient but how much and what kind of transfer occurs during that time.

It was asked whether the patients sometimes feel the doctor withholds information they think they should know. This was an attempt to tackle the communication problem from another angle. Fully 70 percent believed this was true. The reasons for this will not yet be surmised but we will note that over two-thirds of the interviewees felt a void in communication where information was either not willingly offered or not furnished (not forthcoming).

The remaining questions sought to measure the general evaluation of medical service—including the linguistic element without setting it apart. Fifty-three percent said they get their money's worth out of medical services, but 57 percent felt doctors are overpaid. When compared with the 25 percent who are in general dissatisfied with the situation (excluding all consideration for operations, medications, and prescriptions), we note, however, that a quarter of the interviewees feel they should be content with what they get even though they do not like the situation as it now stands, while an additional quarter are still not appeased by the benefits of their medical attention at all.

Thus, the pilot survey of patient reactions to their communication problems with doctors yields rather clear results. In almost every case, about half the respondents expressed some sort of evidence of communication failure in the medical interview. One can always question the validity of self-report data of this sort, for it is difficult to determine how accurate the patients' responses really were. The conditions under which this survey was conducted, however, are such that one might expect the patients to be somewhat intimidated into denying communciation failure rather than admitting it, particularly since they were asked these questions in the hospital waiting rooms.

DO ACTUAL MEDICAL INTERVIEWS OFFER
EVIDENCE OF COMMUNICATION BREAKDOWN?

Far better than asking patients outright whether or not they feel that there is a communication problem in the medical interview is the technique of actually observing such problems in real life settings.* To this point, my colleagues and I have tape recorded over one hundred such interviews.

Earlier we stated that we were interested in determining the extent to which the medical history is conducted on a continuum from doctor language to patient language. By far, the largest parts of the medical interviews were conducted in doctor language and the patients tried very hard to operate in as close a version of doctor language as they could muster. Most serious breakdowns came when patients could (or would) not speak doctor language and doctors could (or would) not understand patient language. Our data, though still brief, display evidences of success and failure at all points on the continuum. The following discussion is presented in the form of a language learning framework, for it appears very clear that the medical interview involves such learning on the part of doctor and patient alike.

Patients Learning to Speak Doctor Talk

Some patients apparently spoke or tried to speak doctor language in order to be accepted or to establish some sort of status with the doctor. A person who can use the terms *mesial* or *distal* to his dentist for example, can feel that he is almost an insider to the dentistry business, even legitimizing his presence in the chair. Some of our patients made very clear and conscientious efforts to speak a language which they judged appropriate for the medical interview. The fact that most of the patients were Black women from inner-city Washington, D.C., would suggest that their gearing-up for the interview would cause them to produce their

---

*It should be made clear that proper authorization was obtained from the hospital administration, from each doctor, and from each patient before such observations were made. In fact, each patient signed a release slip permitting us to tape record the medical interview for the purpose of research.

best formal English, as free as possible from stigmatized grammatical features. The patients generally guarded against the use of vernacular English by offering relatively short and formal responses, slipping only in utterances which might be considered non-medical or near social, such as:

D: Does Mr. Jones work?
P: He *work* manually. He *work* at the courthouse downtown.

or in hypercorrections such as:

P: Well, I just had infection, you know—a *kidneys* infection.

or in emotional circumstances such as the description of intense pain as follows:

D: And what's the chest pain like?
P: They don't really stay in one place. They *comes* right up in here. Then *it* goes round the side, then, you know, just up and down and round the side.
D: Ever under your arm?
P: Yes, in this arm here and it, and like when I wake up, I *can't hardly* hold it, you know, it go to sleep. It's all pain here—hurts—and then when I wake up I *can't hardly* close my joints—so stiff.
D: Is this—does it hurt?
P: Yeah, and then I, you know, when I try to use it, it *feel* like it goes dead and *don't have no* feeling in it.

The shorter emergency room interviews tended to be more fraught with frantic emotion, yielding little guarding against vernacular such as:

P: Look, I *ain't gonna sign* . . .
D: Is this your first or last (name)?
P: *That* my first. *Arnold* my last.
D: Your nose stuffed up?
P: Not my nose, It my body.

P: I tell you where I *comes* from it never rain.

Most generally during the major portions of the medical interview, however, very little vernacular Black English was employed by the patients, despite every indication that such a vernacular is habitual in more formal contexts. This suggests that they were putting on their best English for the occasion, a fact which in itself suggests that they were attempting to speak doctor talk.

Occasionally doctor talk was actually learned during the interview:

> D: And have you ever had any accidents, breaking an arm, break a leg . . .?
>
> P: Not broken, but, I, when your arm is in a sling that means it's not broken. It's not always knocked out of place, but this was when I was a child.
>
> D: It was dislocated.
>
> P: Well, right, dislocated, OK? (nervous laughter)

Another instance of this learning can be seen on another occasion when a woman who had had six previous pregnancies learned the sequence and language of responding very quickly:

> D: OK, now your second child?
>
> P: 1959, Georgetown, normal pregnancy.
>
> D: And how about the, uh, duration of labor?
>
> P: I'd say it was 1:00 when I came here that night and my son was born at 5:30 in the morning—5:30 A.M.—so I guess it must have been around 4 hours.
>
> D: And . . .
>
> P: Normal. They were all six pound babies.

This anticipatory response continued through the descriptions of the other four deliveries as well:

> D: And your fourth child?
>
> P: 1961.
>
> D: Where was she born?
>
> P: Here, the same, and I don't remember.
>
> D: (Laughs) We're getting this down pat now, aren't we?

In addition to the direct teaching of medical terms (as in the case of dislocated arm) and cumulative experience (as in learning the predicted medical history question sequences (immediately preceding), patients also learn to talk doctor language in a rather dangerous manner as a result of intimidation:

> D: You *are* drinking a lot of milk, aren't you?
>
> P: Oh, yes, I drink a lot of milk.

Upon completion of the interview, we overheard the nurse ask the patient the same question and the patient answered, this time truthfully, that she hated milk and never touched it. Why would she lie to the doctor? Probably because the question was asked in such a way that the patient was afraid to answer truthfully.

Another level of intimidation seems to derive less from the doctor's manner than from the obviousness of the question. Somehow we expect ourselves to have perfect memory for certain things like our own telephone numbers, our family's birthdates, and other such matters. Our data reveal several examples of patient embarrassment at such lapses in memory:

D: Now, your first child. . .what year was he born?

P: She was born in 1957.

D: 1957?

P: This is terrible! I have to think.

Equally embarrassing is the patient's general inability to pronounce the names of drugs properly or, in some cases, even to remember them:

D: Chest pains? OK. Do you use any medications?

P: I was on, uh, what you call it? Diagrens—they call Diagr. . .

D: Hmmm. Have you ha. . ., have you taken them during this pregnancy?

P: No.

D: Anything that you've taken during this pregnancy?

P: I had some Dia. . . They gave me some vitamins, some green pills and I had some little, bitty white pills, and some red pills.

This interlude was particularly tender because of the patient's complete failure at speaking doctor talk. She got no reinforcement from the doctor, who may not know what Diagren is either, and, lacking support and realizing defeat, the patient resorted to the total layman, even childish, language of red, green and white pills.

In some cases, clear evidence of a patient's ability to talk doctor language seems apparent:

D: Were there any complications as far as you were concerned?

P: Well, I did have excessive weight gain as I have now and, uh, that was toward the end of the pregnancy and they put me on a salt-free diet.

This exchange came at the very end of the interview, and perhaps evidences the patient's language learning skills, even to the extent of impersonalizing her pregnancy to *the* pregnancy and sprinkling lightly with hospital lingo such as *excessive wieght gain* and *salt-free diet.*

Patients Learning to Understand Doctor Talk

Doctors do not always make it easy for patients to understand them. Occasionally this stems from inexperience or a simple inability to ask questions well. Surprisingly, patients are frequently able to guess at the intention of the question even when it is inelegantly stated:

    D: Now did he have any problems during the pregnancy of the child?

    P: No.

This question follows a discussion of the delivery of the patient's second child during which no antecedent for the he exists. It can only be assumed that the doctor meant *you* for *he*. Likewise, the doctor obviously means *your pregnancy* for *pregnancy of the child*. This was a terribly garbled sentence, yet the patient answered without the slightest hesitation, apparently disambiguating as she went along.

Patients in these interviews were also very consistent in answering multiple questions put forth by doctors. The following multiple questions will serve as examples:

    D: Well, how do you feel? Did you have a fever?

    P: No.

    D: How long have you had that? All your life?

    P: Yes.

    D: Where do you get short of breath? Do you ever wake up short of breath?

    P: No.

    D: And in your family, was there any heart problems—any heart disease? Do you talk to your parents a lot?

    P: Yes.

    D: Did you ever have rheumatic fever? Did you ever have scarlet fever? Break out in a rash?

    P: No.

It can be assumed that the consistency of the patients here in

answering only the last of a multiple questions series is transported from their same question answering strategies used in
other contexts. In the last two examples, the *yes* and *no* cannot
answer the first questions in those examples. This transportation
of regular question answering strategies to the medical history
interview is not surprising from the patient's perspective but it
casts considerable question on the interpretation of the answers.
What indeed will the doctor do with an answer of *yes* to his
question, "How long have you had that?" What will he do with
an answer of *no* to his inquiry, "Where do you get short of
breath?"

On some occasions the doctor's questions are simply not
understood by the patient:

    D: Have you ever had a history of cardiac arrest in your
       family?

    P: We never had no trouble with the police.

    D: What's your name?

    P: Betty Groff.

    D: How do you spell that?

    P: B-E-T-T-Y.

    D: How about varicose veins?

    P: Well, I have veins, but I don't know if they're close or not.

In the analysis of the taped medical histories, however, we were
only infrequently given such clear examples of misunderstanding. There are many other occasions in which one might
seriously question the understanding of the patient on technical
language. In several instances, when the doctor appeared to be
hurrying through his list of diseases and illnesses, we noted what
we are calling negative weakening, as illustrated by the following:

    D: . . . Is there any incidence of high blood pressure?

    P: No. (strongly)

    D: Tuberculosis?

    P: No. (Average stress)

    D: Epilepsy?

    P: No. (weakly)

    D: Neurological or psychological problems?

    P: (shakes head)

D: Allergies?

P: (No response)

That is, the series of technical terms has triggered a negative series in which the response is at first strong (perhaps because the questions are more familiar) but gradually weakens acoustically and finally devoices into negative head shaking. Even stronger evidence for the incomprehensibility of this series of questions can be observed in the very next response in this same interview.

D: Multiple births?

P: (Long pause) I had a retarded child once.

Later in the same interview the patient responded with a strong *no* to German measles, a weak *no* to chronic problems and a head-shaking negation to both vaginitis and cervicitis.

Naturally, some doctors are more sensitive than others to their patients' lack of knowledge of doctor talk. Some attempt to determine what the layman needs to know is made:

Relative: Is he gonna live?

D: Well, are you his wife?

P: Yes.

D: Well, he's had a cardiac arrest. Do you understand what this is?

P: Yeah.

D: Well, he's in very critical condition. We have a tube in him and he has some pressure of his own. So, we'll see him in about a half-hour if there's been any change.

It is doubtful, in this emergency room setting, that the relative would have asked the doctor for an explanation of cardiac arrest. But he might have tried to do a better job than he did. The implication seems to be clear and consistent. Patients and relatives of patients should play the doctor game in the doctor setting, similar to the way Americans expect all foreigners to speak English in our country.

In stark contrast, one hospital doctor actually began his history in the following way:

D: I want to know if you have any questions you might want to ask.

P: No, nothing I can think of.

D: OK, we'll go on from there.

The question undoubtedly took the patient by surprise, for

almost everyone has questions to ask about his health if he is given the opportunity and freedom to ask them. This doctor opened the door, but it may take patients a while to get used to their new role in his office.

As an adjunct to the study of the tape recorded medical histories, we might call upon the data recently extracted from attempts at automated techniques for acquiring medical information. One such application involves the condensation of several basic medical tests into one functional unit called a multiphasic testing facility (or multi-test clinic). The particular series of tests and procedures employed emphasize the differentiation of a general population into two major subgroups: (1) the apparently healthy who require little more than reassurance and periodic status checking and (2) the probably ill who require further evaluation and, in all likelihood, treatment.

A prime discriminator in such a differentiation is the interpretation of the medical history. The patient answers a self-administered series of questions by pressing various buttons on a console. The written questions appear on an illuminated screen and the patient selects from the multiple choice answers. He can take as long as he wants, go back to earlier questions, change answers, leave blanks or call for the nurse to help him interpret a question. All of his answers are recorded electronically within seconds and are organized into a convenient print-out for the physician to interpret at his convenience.

Several things may be criticized in this procedure and it is my intention neither to defend it nor attack it here. Of greater interest to me is the fact that the questions asked were devised by physicians on the basis of their past experience in face-to-face medical interviewing. The content and wording of the questions may be assumed to be representative of the more individualized and time-consuming, patient-doctor communication. The concepts and the language of such questions are clearly middle-class, uninvolved and jargonish and, as such, they offer further evidence of the requirement of patients to learn to talk like doctors. They are seldom close to the inner-city patient's point of view or experience level. Even the briefest overview of such questions will yield areas of concern such as the question-answer categories offered in the answers and the instructions.

1. *The Question-Answer Categories.* In an effort to obtain background information on the kinds of physical activities in which a patient engages, the medical profession takes a clearly middle-class stance. Questions which ask for data on the amount of time spent exercising, for example, have a distinct bourgeois ring to them (jogging, tennis, skiing). Most inner-city residents walk at least 20 minutes a day and would find the question unnecessary. It may be possible to eliminate this sort of question for certain audiences but, at least, the alternatives should be modified to activities which are more real to them. Such a question is culturally equivalent to asking them whether they read *The Wall Street Journal, The New York Times,* or *Atlantic.*

2. *The Range of Choice Offered in Answers.* Occasionally wording is potentially unclear to any audience. For example, "How do you feel about your work?" This is very close to what linguists might call a stereotype question. That is, if asked, "How are you?", most people would answer, "Fine," regardless of their present state of health. The temptation is to answer a stereotype question with a stereotype answer. The whole interchange performs a social function rather than an intellectual one. A question about work is made even muddier, however, by the word *feel,* which could trigger any number of possible responses. If such a question is to be preserved in the examination, care must be taken to find cultural equivalents to the rather middle-class responses.

In one question, a male patient was asked what his main reason was for seeing the doctor. There are few working-class men who will admit to having an emotional problem. However accurate the term might be, it is not likely to be employed by a man whose status and livelihood are dependent on his masculinity. Emotional problems indicate weakness. It is easier to admit being injured than sick. Again, research will have to determine the best wording to trigger the desired response. At this time, it is difficult to tell.

Not only is patient-doctor communication affected by the language and culture of the doctor, but also by the culture of the patient. Zborowski studied the reactions to pain of various New York City ethnic groups and concluded that while Jewish and Italian-Americans responded to pain quite emotionally, more assimilated Americans were more objective and stoical, and Irish-Americans more frequently even denied the existence of pain.[11] Furthermore, Italian-Americans were usually satisfied when relief from pain was obtained while Jewish patients were mainly concerned about the underlying meaning of pain and its potential consequences for their future well-being. Mechanic[7] notes that this study and others of the same type do not clarify whether such ethnic differences and upbringing have more objective symptoms, interpret the same symptoms differently, express their problems more willingly, more eagerly seek help or use a different vocabulary for expressing distress. It is important that such distinctions be researched.

The effect of social learning on the language system of ill or probably ill people is carefully observed by Zborowski,[11] who points out that in "old American" families, the mother teaches her children to endure pain "like a man" and to avoid crying. If a doctor is consulted, it should be for physical, not psychological distress. Likewise, Zola[12] studied the evaluations by doctors of patients from various ethnic groups for whom no medical disease was found. He found that Italians, who were more emotional in the presentation of symptoms and gave more attention to the expression of pain and stress, were more likely to be diagnosed as suffering from a psychogenic condition than were members of other ethnic groups. Similarly, Bart[1] observed that women who were admitted on a neurology service and were diagnosed as having psychiatric disorders were less educated, more rural, of lower socioeconomic status, and less likely to be Jewish than women who entered a hospital for psychiatric help directly. Bart further noted that the two groups of women were differentiated by their vocabularies of complaint, which obviously affected the manner in which they presented themselves. The ultimate consequences of expressing psychologic distress through physical attribution can be seen in Bart's follow-up study in which 52 percent of the psychiatric patients on the neurology service had hysterectomies while only 21 percent of the women who went directly to psychiatric treatment had such surgery, suggesting that patients who express psychologic distress through physical attributions expose themselves to apparently unnecessary medical procedures.

The general impression resulting from such studies as those of Zborowski, Mechanic, and Bart is that at least two major patterns of patient behavior may mislead the physician as he attempts to obtain verbal information relating to their medical history.

1. The patient who is willing to use the vocabulary of physical and psychologic distress, complaining openly and admitting frustration and unhappiness. Such a patient may seem hypochondriacal but she is at least not culture-bound to distort or hide her symptoms or problems.

2. The more difficult (and more common) patient who, for whatever reason (including cultural background), has a different vocabulary for reporting distress from that of the physician.

Of these two patterns, Mechanic observes that the second group

> ...present the doctor with a variety of diffuse physical complaints for which he can find no clear-cut explanation, but he cannot be sure that they do not indeed suffer from some physical disorder that he has failed to diagnose. Patients who express psychologic distress through a physical language tend to be uneducated or come from cultural groups where the expression of emotional distress is either inhibited or different from middle class norms. Such patients frequently face serious life difficulties and social stress, but the subculture within which they function does not allow legitimate expression of their suffering nor are others attentive to their pleas for support when they are made. Because of their experiences these patients frequently feel...that expression of their difficulties is a sign of weakness and will be deprecated. They thus dwell on bodily complaints....[7]

Medical specialists will need to learn that questions involving expressions such as an *infection like pneumonia* or *blood poisoning* are middle-class analogies. Many people do not think of pneumonia as an infection. Likewise for many people, *diabetes* is less likely to be understood than *sugar* or *sugar diabetes*, and *heart disease* is more likely to be recognized as *heart trouble*. In such cases as the latter, it may be true that patients can respond to the stimulus *heart disease* even though they use the term *heart trouble*. But we do not know, as yet, if even this is true. In any case, problems involving the heart are not generally thought of as *disease* in the working-class community. It has been hypothesized that *heart attack* is recognized as that which kills a person who may or may not have a history of problems with his heart, while *heart trouble* indicates a history of the disease. Such information, if true, could be helpful in a technical way which is, at present, untapped by the medical profession. There are, in addition, many other everyday terms used by ghetto residents which could be employed in such a questionnaire. *Consumption*, for example, in inner-city Washington, D.C., is used in reference to a person who drinks himself to death. *Diarrhea* is more commonly known as *runny bowels* or *running off at the bowels.*

The doctor's over-use of his technical language tends to estrange him from the patient by setting himself on a much higher intellectual level. This may inhibit the patient in his communication—e.g., fear of asking questions that the doctor might consider stupid or superfluous. One patient received the following typed physician's report from the clinic where she was examined:

BARIUM ENEMA WITH AIR CONTRAST:
There is normal filling and evacuation of the colon.
There is reflux into the terminal ileum which appears
normal. There are multiple nontender diverticula,
predominantly involving the descending colon and
sigmoid portion of the colon. No other abnormalities
are identified. Incidentally noted is calcification
within the uterine fibroids in the true pelvis.
This was the only information she received on her medical condition.

Doctors Learning to Understand Patient Talk

It will take considerably more data than are now available for us to catalogue the types of misunderstandings doctors have of patient language, primarily because the patient says so little during the medical history, following a strategy so successfully used by minority school children who learn very early that the name of the game is to be right as often as possible and wrong as seldom as possible and that the best way to avoid being wrong is to keep one's mouth shut. Another reason why we have so few examples of doctor's misunderstanding of patient language stems from the social structure of the speech event. The doctor is simply not to be wrong. If anyone is wrong, it is the patient. Still a third reason for the paucity of evidence on doctors' misunderstanding of patient talk stems from the feedback system. There seems to be no immediate way to determine how he has actually misassessed the validity of the patient's *no* when, in truth, the answer is *yes*. We have already cited a fortuitous example of two of such evidence, but such proof is hard to come by.

We have recorded an instance, however, in which clear acquisition of patient talk by a doctor seems to have taken place:

P: Oh, he did, uh, in last April he had a little touch of sugar when...

D: He has a little what?

P: You know, diabetic...

D: Oh, he had some sugar.

A more serious example occurred during an early observation during which the doctor asked the patient if she had ever had an abortion. She denied that she had, even though her chart clearly indicated two previous abortions. In the doctor's mind, the patient had chosen to tell a lie for the evidence was clearly before him. After the doctor had left, the patient was asked by a linguist whether or not she had ever lost a baby. She readily admitted to having lost two. In the ensuing conversation it was determined that the patient was defining abortion as self-induced while the doctor was using the term to refer to a wider range of possibilities. It seems obvious here that the doctor has not learned the patient's language.

Doctors Learning to Speak Patient Talk

If evidence from our research and from the accounts in medical literature is accurate, few doctors have mastered the ability to speak the language of the working class, minority, or foreign-language-speaking patient. Severe problems can result from miscommunication on all levels, particularly for the non-English speaker. In fact, the clearest mandate seems to be for hospitals, clinics, and other medical facilities to gear up for medical services for speakers of foreign languages.

A more cautious note must be sounded, however, for the need for doctors to attempt to speak patient dialect, a practice which can lead to serious problems. For example, one conscientious doctor, sensitive to the fact that his patient was Black and poor, assumed that she would be more comfortable with homey expressions, despite the fact that she had already passed through such fine distinctions as phlebitis, rheumatic fever, transfusions, and epilepsy. He was doing very well in his interview, giving the appearance of casual yet professional ease. He was friendly and interested in the patient as a person. And then he blew it with his liberal enthusiasm:

D: What about belly pain?

P: (Pause, followed by recovery) No.

D: (Unperturbed and growing more dramatic) Have you had a problem with burning when you urinate or do you find you're running to the john every five minutes?

P: (Slowly) No.

D: (With increasing loudness) Or do you have an extreme urgency, like do you feel when you have to go urinate that, Oh, the urge is just tremendous that you have to run and get there or else you'll wet your pants?

If these questions seem ludicrous to us, how much more ludicrous must they have seemed to the patient. Here she was, working desperately to speak doctor talk, with medical terminology and a minimum of vernacular grammar and he uses words like *belly, john,* and *wet your pants.* The effect must be similar to that of a 55-year-old youth worker trying to talk teenage slang. It is also akin to the problem some of us have who grew up speaking a nonstandard dialect but, having gotten educated, are no longer allowed to use it by the people we grew up with and love. Their expectation of us simply will not allow it even though they may continue to use it themselves.

WHAT IS THE LANGUAGE OF THE MEDICAL HISTORY?

As noted earlier, by far the largest part of the medical history, from the data available to us so far, indicates a doctor dominance in language and perspective. It is, in one sense at least, his native country, his home grounds. The patient is the foreigner or intruder. A great deal has been said in recent years about a similar situation in education. For a long time we have made noises about starting with the child where he is and yet, as mentioned earlier, massive programs have been mounted to remake children in the eyes of the school norm so that they can benefit from the teaching perspective. Such programs are saying, in effect, that the child is simply not good enough, and that in order to be taught he must become like the school, especially in matters of language and culture. It appears that a similar situation obtains in medicine. Our limited data show that about half of the patients surveyed feel extremely uncomfortable about understanding what doctors are telling them and about making themselves clear to doctors. An equal number feel that doctors are generally unfriendly and intimidating. Our tape recorded data reveal startling instances to verify the communication breakdown and call to question the efficiency of the medical interview in cross-cultural settings. Add to this the fact that it is the patient who is at the disadvantage. She is either in need of medical attention or thinks she has such a need. Just as one might expect a person with education to adjust to the needs of the person being taught, so might one expect the healthy to adjust to the needs of the sick. And yet, strong indication exists that such an adjustment is only infrequently made. With the exceptions of the histories taken by the private physicians in our study, we can safely generalize that the doctors do not speak patient language and, much more seriously, that they often give little evidence of trying to understand it. The patient generally adjusts to the doctor's perspective, actually offering medical terms whenever possible. When the patient cannot do this well, the history is slowed and made less efficient. In short, the general expectation is for the patient to learn doctor talk.

A great deal could be learned by the clinic doctors from the technique of one physician whose demeanor was relaxed, congenial and enthusiastic. Some random quotations from his histories will serve as examples:

...Here's an illustration of what I mean.
...Great! It'll probably work out fine for you.
...Let's watch that but don't worry too much about it.
...You look like a million dollars.
...Mrs. M, are there any questions I can answer for you?
...No problems here. And your last labor was much too easy.
...So what I'd like to say is that everything that's going on is quite normal.

It may take a long time for this doctor's patients to learn to take advantage of the openings he regularly provides them to ask any question they want. One of his patients confided:

I thought he was too busy so I didn't ask a lot of things

until I was in my ninth month. Then Dr. G. realized that I, you know, had been holding back. But we got everything straightened out in time.

This same doctor evidenced a clear appreciation of the language needs of his patients. Although he never attempted to speak vernacular Black English himself (fully realizing how ludicrous it might sound), he was sensitive to his obligation to help the patient understand his language, without being patronizing or stuffy. For example, to a sixteen year old patient he said:

Incidentally, Ann, you might have noticed that you have a lot of mucus and that's normal...and it's called leukorrhea.

The approach was not, "You have leukorrhea." Such a statement would either require the patient to ask what the term means, thus lowering her status even further or to retreat to fearful and ignorant silence, a strategy which I suspect to be frequent in our data.

In summary, of the general points on the doctor—patient, medical history language continuum the major breakdowns occur at the extremes. Some patients cannot or will not speak doctor language. Likewise, some doctors cannot or will not speak patient language. It has been suggested, in fact, that it is probably disastrous for them to try. The obvious area of hope lies in the central portions of the continuum.

APPENDIX A: QUESTIONNAIRE

	Yes	No
1. Do you ever feel that when doctors, nurses or interns ask you questions they sometimes use words that are hard to understand?	___	___
2. Do you ever find the doctor's attitude unfriendly?	___	___
3. Do you ever find it hard to make the doctor understand what a pain is like or where it is?	___	___
4. Do you think the doctor spends enough time talking with you during an appointment?	___	___

before an operation? _____ _____

after an operation? _____ _____

5. Do you think nurses or hospital assistants pay enough attention to your needs when you are in the hospital? _____ _____

6. Do you think that medical people expect you to know too many medical words? _____ _____

7. Do you ever feel that sometimes you do not want to ask a doctor a question because he might think it is stupid? _____ _____

8. Do you think doctors get too much money for what they do? _____ _____

9. Do you think that doctors should spend more time talking with you than they do? _____ _____

10. Do you ever think that the doctor does not understand your problem? _____ _____

11. Do you think sometimes that doctors should speak in more simple language? _____ _____

12. Do you ever feel that doctors do not tell you everything you should know about a problem, condition or an operation? _____ _____

13. Do you think you get your money's worth when you go for medical advice, checkups or other medical problems? _____ _____

14. In general, are you satisfied with the kind of medical attention you get besides actual operations, medications and prescriptions? _____ _____

REFERENCES

1. P. B. Bart, Social structure and vocabularies of discomfort: what happened to female hysteria? *J Health Soc Behav,* 9:188-93, 1968.
2. D. L. Brazelon, At last psychiatry must open its doors. *Los Angeles Times,* July 1, 1976.
3. A. V. Cicourel, Interviewing and memory. To appear in a special issue of *Theory and Decision.*
4. A. Hollingshead and F. Redlich, *Social Class and Mental Illness.* New York: John Wiley & Sons, 1958.
5. D. Hymes, The contribution of folklore to sociolinguistic research. *J Am Folklore,* 84, 1971.

6. C. P. Kimball, Medicine and dialects. *Ann Intern Med*, 74:137-139, 1971.
7. D. Mechanic, Some psychologic factor affecting the presentation of bodily complaints. *New Engl J Med*, 286:1132-39, 1972.
8. D. Robinson, 10 noted doctors answer 10 tough questions. *Parade*, July 15, 1973.
9. R. W. Shuy, Sociolinguistics and the medical history. Paper presented at the Third International Conference on Applied Linguistics (Copenhagen), 1974.
10. B. Stoeltje, *History Taking*, Unpublished manuscript, The University of Texas, 1971.
11. M. Zborowski, Cultural components of response to pain. *J Soc Issues*, 8:16-30, 1952.
12. I. K. Zola, Problems of communication, diagnosis, and patient care: the interplay of patient, physician and clinic organization. *J Med Educ*, 38:822-38, 1963.

PROBLEM-ORIENTED APPROACH TO EXTENDED MEDICAL INTERVIEW

THOMAS WOLMAN

A successful medical interview evolves happily for both doctor and patient. There is a free flow of information and a sense of partnership in which both parties work to open areas of inquiry. Doctor and patient have a sense of satisfaction and closure when the interview ends.

It is especially discouraging when this expected result does not occur. All too often, some disturbance in communication supervenes early in an interview, leading to stalemate and shared frustration. In the extreme case, dialogue degenerates into interrogation.

This paper will attempt to highlight some problems in interviewing and present strategies for re-establishing successful communication through problem solving. Standard history taking and interview technique will not be reviewed. We see our remarks as being applicable to any extended medical interview.

Data for this project consisted in part of videotapes of extended medical interviews done by students at Jefferson Medical College.

COMMUNICATION

We hypothesize that communication and data gathering should not be considered as separate processes. Overcoming blocks in communication not only enhances rapport but increases knowledge. As an illustration consider the following vignette:

From Thomas Wolman, Problem-Oriented Approach to Extended Medical Interview, *Pennsylvania Medicine*, 82:27-30,1979. Courtesy of Pennsylvania Medical Society.

A young healthy-looking man is being interviewed, with the chief complaint that he is bringing up excess phlegm. What is the urgency of seeing a physician for this now? Early on, the patient says that past x-rays revealed "a spot on the lung...the tongue...I guess maybe it was my throat." The doctor assumes it was in the throat and proceeds with the interview which quickly shifts to a discussion of fatty tissue in the patient's right thigh. Only later in the interview does it become clear that there was a spot on the lung and that tuberculosis was suspected.

If the doctor in the above case had shifted away from history taking and instead focused attention on the patient's contradictory ambiguous statement, the outcome might have been different. A critical piece of information could have been established earlier, thus helping to direct further inquiry.

PROBLEMS OF THE OPENING PHASE

The opening phase of an interview is as critical as the opening move of a chess game. Communication problems are most frequent in this phase, and they have the most disturbing effect on the course of the interview. The following three problem areas represent key difficulties:

1. *Failure to adequately explore the chief complaint.* A full exploration of the chief complaint is essential for the proper development of the interview. This involves eliciting details which comprise a complete picture of the context in which the chief complaint occurs. The most frequent error seen in interviewing is a premature shift from work on the chief complaint to consideration of other topics. The following vignette is illustrative:

A 25-year-old man mentions anxiety attacks as the chief complaint. He casually mentions that the first attack occurred after his girl friend of seven years left him. At this point the interviewer abruptly shifts to questions about alcohol intake, appetite, etc. Finally, after consultation with an instructor, the interviewer returns to the chief complaint. Unexpectedly the patient now reports a second symptom: an automobile phobia which might have been missed.

The most devastating consequence of the premature shift is the doctor's feeling of disorientation. This usually occurs in the middle of the interview. Without a full picture of the chief complaint as a beacon, the interviewer reaches a point where he is insecure and does not know what to ask. At this point he may flounder and blindly ask any question which comes to mind. As the above vignette shows, the best remedy is to drop everything and return to the chief complaint.

Perfunctory work on the chief complaint also may lead to misunderstanding. As part of the examination, we should ask the patient to tell us specifically how he experiences the complaint. This often will clear up ambiguities. For instance, some patients say they are anxious when they mean depressed, or paranoid when they mean anxious. This is related to the relaxed use of certain terms in common speech. Other patients present the chief complaint as a kind of password for initiating the interview when in fact their reason for being there is entirely different.* The following vignette considers some of these difficulties:

A 25-year-old woman begins the interview by stating that, "I think I have a death wish." She then begins to talk of unrelated problems at work. We can notice immediately the extreme ambiguity of the chief complaint. Does it mean that the patient is depressed? Self-destructive? Incidentally, the form of the chief complaint is often a good clue to the patient's inner life and worthy of exploration in itself. In this case it was perfectly characteristic of this patient's tendency to use intellectual abstraction to convey her emotional concerns.

2. *Failure to diagnose the communicational style of the patient.* Many people have a rather fixed notion of the role of the interviewer—the triad of sitting back passively, listening and asking general open-ended questions. This strategy will fail completely with many types of patients. Early in an interview we must ask the question, "How is this patient communicating with me?" We must conduct the interview on the basis of what the patient can accomplish and what will be practical to get the interview moving. If we discover that open-ended questions yield

---

* In a small proportion of interviews, the chief complaint is absent entirely. In these situations it is doubly important to ascertain why the patient wants to talk.

no response, we must shift tactics. Table IV-1 is an attempt to match specific strategies with over-all communications styles. Table IV-2 is an attempt to deal with the language style of patients from lower socioeconomic classes who may not be able or willing to play the language game of the formal interview.

3. *Failure to deal with disturbances in the working alliance.* At a certain point in the opening phase it is essential to ask, "Is this patient ready to work together with me?" In other words, is there a sense of communicational give-and-take? If the answer is yes, we can proceed to the body of the interview. If the answer is no, something must be done if the interview is not to become a one-sided no-information affair.

Usually the reason for a shaky working alliance is anxiety or anger on the part of the patient as the following vignette will illustrate:

> A young woman says her chief complaint is intense fear of people, especially those she first meets. At this point the interviewer must assume that such anxiety is occurring then and there. If he simply proceeds with the questioning, he will be faced by a frightened, taciturn patient. He could handle the problem by inquiring if the patient is anxious now, and if so, whether they can talk about it. As anxiety decreases, dialogue continues.

PROBLEMS OF THE MIDDLE PHASE

With the successful completion of the opening phase, an interviewer often experiences a smooth, almost effortless transition to the body of the interview. The problems encountered here are not incapacitating (as are the ones in the first phase). Rather, they relate to the deepening of the interview process and the acceleration of data gathering. Concentrated listening by the doctor is important, both to pick up concealed information and help select the best track to follow. We select four problems for detailed discussion.

1. *Deflection away from the patient's emotional focus.* If the patient begins to explore emotionally laden areas spontaneously, it is best not to interfere. Consider the following situation.:

> A 28-year-old married woman was talking about her bad marriage and her fear of going crazy. Later, with much affect,

TABLE IV-1

INTERVIEW STRATEGIES BASED ON THE PATIENT'S COMMUNICATIONAL STYLE

Communicational Style	Common Interviewer Errors	Consequences of Errors	Sample Strategy
Taciturn	Higher frequency of non-stop questions	Limited data; experience of pulling teeth	a. Focus on patient's reticence; b. Negotiate for mutually acceptable neutral area.
Loquacious with pressured speech	Passive stance	Limited data; loss of control of interview	a. Partial structuring of interview; b. Bringing patient back to areas glossed over; c. Confronting patient, "I can't get a word in edgewise."
Open, verbal, psychologically minded	Too many yes-no questions	Intensity of interview is damped	Ask open-ended questions and let patient tell own story.
Concrete (i.e., mildly organic)	Open-ended and abstract questions asked ("Tell me about yourself.")	Patient blocks on these questions and interview grinds to a halt.	a. Lead patient through specific situations; b. Ask him to role-play what he and others would say in this situation.
Disorganized (i.e., due to psychosis)	Passive stance; concentrated attempt to get coherent story	Limited data; loss of control of interview; frustration of interviewer.	a. Shortened interview; b. Deal with affect expressed; c. Defer history.
Intellectual and abstract	Passive stance; open-ended, general questions; failure to concretize or personalize material.	Affects remain hidden; limited data.	a. Ask more specific questions; b. Comment on affects; c. Ask for examples; d. Ask patient to personalize concepts.

TABLE IV-2
PROBLEMS AND TACTICAL PLAN FOR INTERVIEWING A PATIENT FROM
A LOWER SOCIOECONOMIC BACKGROUND

Problem	Tactic
Patient may not elaborate on a general question, i.e., "Tell me about your home life."	a. Ask specific questions. Lead patient through a "guided tour" of his home and family; b. Use modified role play. Ask "What would your father say?" and "What would you then say?"
Patient may not take measure to make sure the correct message is getting across to interviewer (metacommunication).	Repeat questions. Clear up ambiguous areas before proceeding.
Patient may not comment on his subjective states or reflect on his own behavior.	a. Focus on patient's external behavior and how he comes across to others; b. Arrange for videotape to be made so the patient can observe himself on television.
The individual may not make explicit subtle aspects of his social code and what is expected in certain situations.	Ask patient to explain these things to you from the point of someone who is especially informed.
Much meaning may be expressed via non-verbal communications, i.e., hand movements, intonation, stress, etc.	Listen carefully and occasionally make explicit what is being expressed non-verbally.

she brought up the subject of her mother's nervous breakdown. At this point the interviewer deflected attention to the patient's brother and sister. Allowing the patient to discuss her mother would have allowed for ventilation of feeling, significant past history and greater comprehension, i.e., a possible connection with the chief complaint.

Physicians frequently are concerned by delving too deeply. A helpful guideline here is that when the patient mentions an emotional issue, he is implicitly telling us, "I am ready to talk about this." If the doctor can listen without shutting the door, the patient may become dramatically less anxious.

2. *Reluctance to focus on here-and-now behavior.* The way a patient behaves in the interview is an immediate here-and-now communication. Such communications directly demonstrate a message, much like a game of charades. Directing attention to

here-and-now behavior often will provide critical information that helps to clear up gaps and inconsistencies in the patient's story. Consider the following material:

> A young woman (referred to above) was being evaluated for intense interpersonal anxiety. In the middle of the interview she abruptly went from relative calm to tears and vague suicidal thoughts. After allowing her to compose herself, the interviewer continued his previous line of questioning. Not following up on this affect shift left gaps in our understanding of the patient. What was she expressing about herself and what were the diagnostic implications? Only further evaluation could tell.

Further examples of here-and-now behavior can be drawn from the full repertoire of nonverbal behavior during the interview. One patient played with her hair throughout an entire interview. This fact became so obvious to the patient that she began to discuss it spontaneously. Information derived from such behavior can act as a check on other information derived from standard history taking. If the patient's actions contradict what he says, we cannot take the history at face value and must investigate further.

3. *Blindness to red flags.* Occasionally the patient will say something at an interview that demands immediate attention. One has no choice but to drop everything and to shift focus to the "red flag" message. A common example is the patient who very casually mentions in the middle of an interview his intention to commit suicide. Needless to say, we do not ignore this, even if the patient attempts to make light of it. Some red flags are not so easy to see, as in the following example:

> In one interview the patient, a young woman, answered all questions and gave her history in a comprehensive manner. However, there was one sharply discordant note: a frantic, desperate, angry tone pervaded all that she said. This affect was a red flag. The confirmation came only when it was ignored and the patient expressed a desire not to return for subsequent interviews.

4. *Problems of pacing and transition in the interview.* As previously mentioned, we allow the pace of the interview to be influenced by feedback from the patient. As we approach the primary emotional focus, we give the lion's share of interview

time. It cannot be stressed too often that preconceived sequences of questions followed relentlessly can ruin the development of the interview. Such lists lead to abrupt transitions which can jar the patient and close off communication. A good interview should unfold or open up. The following vignettes illustrate the timing of transitions:

> The patient with fear of people mentions that she fears people are talking about her. At this point the interviewer smoothly introduces a mental status exam inquiring about auditory hallucinations and other perceptual distortions.

> An angry young woman feels she is treated in a hostile, demeaning manner. After citing a long list of abuses, she mentions that her father, with whom she previously had been close, had rejected her after she had had an abortion. At this point the interviewer asks about the father, opening up the topic of past family history.

In an unfolding interview, various relevant topics should emerge from the immediate context, without sacrificing completeness.

PROBLEMS OF THE CLOSING PHASE

In this stage the physician faces the challenge of consolidating his understanding of the patient and ending the interview in a manner which is not traumatic for the patient. Three aspects of closing will be merely touched upon here.

1. *Untraumatic termination.* Usually the interviewer can establish the working alliance for future interviews by outlining and defining a closing phase which gives the patient time to adjust to separation. We can ask if the patient has any questions which we have not discussed. Most importantly, we must make some kind of statement to the patient. This statement may communicate: (a.) our partial understanding of what is going on with the patient, (b.) our assurance that we have recognized the patient's distress and will work with him in doing something about it, and (c.) reassurance, at times, that the patient's problem is treatable. This statement often is omitted because of anxiety generated by the patient's urgent query, "What is wrong with me?" We want to emphasize that an exact answer is not necessary

(especially since we may not know), but that some response is required.

2. *Covert messages and counter transference.* It is useful for the doctor to ask himself, "What is this patient implicitly telling me?" or "What is this patient implicitly appealing to me to do?" A methodical spelling out of how the interviewer felt during the interview may provide clues to the covert message. Such knowledge may help orient the interviewer in the future. The following example is representative:

A 40-year-old unmarried school teacher is worried that she may kill a child. In an embittered tone she launches into a harangue against the school and principal. The theme is clearly summarized as "I have broken my back, and look what they have done for me." Consequently the appeal to the the interviewer is "Look at all I have been through; please give me some sympathy." If the doctor has not articulated this message in his mind, he may simply experience a countertransference reaction of feeling sorry for the patient. If he is not aware of this reaction, he may act on it, perhaps giving the patient excessive reassurance. This in turn may yield a distorted picture of the patient in subsequent interviews.

CONCLUSIONS AND A NOTE

This approach to the extended medical interview was shaped by the practical necessities of teaching medical students interviewing skills. Instead of telling doctors to do A, B, and C, we have found it most useful to define technique negatively. One begins, and then somewhere along the line a problem occurs which impedes progress. We teach a technique which identifies problems at whatever phase they occur and goes on to formulate strategies for their resolution. Incidentally, not much has been said positively about the interviewer's collection of interventions.

Since this would comprise a paper in itself, we would only note the following: In line with what has been said, it is critical that the interviewer not fall into the rut in which questions are his only form of intervention. This only will tend to close up the interview, yielding only literal answers to the questions. The range of possible alternatives to questions is really as large as that in ordinary animated conversation. It includes everything from exclamations to requests, comments and interpretations.

The problem-oriented approach presupposes several general rules. It stresses the ordering of priorities in the interview by accomplishing the most pressing tasks first. A corollary to this could be called Sutton's law of the interview: Always deal with the patient's primary emotional focus first (go where the money is). Also, a certain mental flexibility is required in order for the interviewer to be ready to change track frequently. Finally, and most importantly, one must be receptive on a moment-to-moment basis to feedback from the patient as the ultimate indication of what to pursue.

REFERENCES

1. H. S. Sullivan, *The Psychiatric Interview*. New York: W. W. Norton, 1954.
2. R. A. Makinnon and R. Michels, *The Psychiatric Interview in Clinical Practice*. Philadelphia: W. B. Saunders, 1971.
3. B. B. Bernstein, *Language and Socialization in Linguistics at Large*. New York: Viking Press, 1971.
4. M. Buber, *The Knowledge of Man: A Philosophy of the Interviewer*. New York: Harper & Row, 1965.
5. M. Balint, *The Doctor, His Patient and the Illness*. New York: International University Press, 1957.

Chapter 5

THE DOCTOR'S TOUCH: TACTILE COMMUNICATION IN THE DOCTOR-PATIENT RELATIONSHIP

JOHN G. BRUHN

Tactile communication is an important aspect of close, personal relationships and is essential in the formation of a doctor-patient relationship, which come under critical scrutiny by both laymen and health professionals. Physicians, in general, are strong advocates of the one-to-one relationship and resist changes in the methods of delivering health care that might alter this relationship. Of particular importance to the physician is the retention of control and decision making in the relationship. Laymen view the problems of the doctor-patient relationship as related more to communication as symbolized by the amount of knowledge they have of each other as persons, and the doctor's performing the expected activities of a clinical examination.

Laying on of the hands in some manner by the doctor is expected by most patients. It is my contention that tactile communication has decreased in the doctor-patient relationship and that this is a source of dissatisfaction for patients. Instrumentation has altered the mode of conducting a clinical examination and has minimized touching of the patient by the physician. New types of health professionals such as physician assistants and nurse practitioners conduct clinical examinations under physician supervision; thus the physician may not "touch" the patient. The type of practice setting may alter a patient's chances of being seen and "touched" by the same physician. These factors are responsible, in part, for diminishing tactile

Reprinted by permission from *The Southern Medical Journal*, (71:1469-73, 1978).

communication between doctor and patient.

The purposes of the present paper are to review the historical meanings of tactile communication to the doctor (the diagnostic touch) and to the patient (the healing touch) and to discuss the importance of touching in the context of changing medical technology.

The skin is an important organ of communication. It exchanges messages between a person's internal and external environments and serves as a thermostat which conveys the nature of the relationships between the two environments. The skin is also an organ of expression of emotion. It receives the direct impact of the environment which it mediates to the organism. The organism interprets the external message and experiences it affectively as emotion.[1] The skin communicates emotion through its color, temperature, and texture. These nonverbal signals together with those from hands, arms, face, touch, stance, and, indeed, the whole body convey meanings which transcend native tongues and culture's speech.

The skin facilitates communication between two or more individuals through touch. The sensory elements of touch induce neural, glandular, muscular and mental changes, which in combination are called emotion. Touch is experienced affectively as emotion. Touch can convey recognition, empathy, and security on the one hand, or anger and hostility on the other. Montagu[2] notes that an infant's first perceptions of reality are through the skin, and adequate tactile satisfaction during infancy and childhood is of fundamental importance for subsequent healthy behavior. He states, for example, that premature babies do better when mothers are allowed to handle them. In his earliest experiences the infant has a number of tactile experiences: close body contacts, being cuddled or patted, touching his lips to his mother's nipple and fingering her breast. The infant evokes from the mother the tactile stimulation which he "needs" and to which he responds in his own fashion. Babies differ widely in their "needs" for tactile experiences and in their acceptance of them. Babies take cues from their mother's behavior as patients take cues from their doctor's behavior. Frank[3] points out that the hands and fingers are like antennae or feelers, a type of feedback mechanism, which probe the surroundings for ensuing motor activities. Each of us learns a highly personal code for communicating, receiving, and interpreting messages from the world and from other persons.

Investigators are paying increasing attention to the intuitive ability of people to pick up and use "expressive" cues in the language and behavior of others, and to the importance of these cues and clues to personality and feeling states. Milmoe and her colleagues,[4] for example, studied the tone and content of doctors' speech as they encountered alcoholics in a hospital emergency room. They found a relationship between an angry tone in the doctor's voice and his lack of effectiveness in referring alcoholics to the special services of the hospital's alcoholic clinic.[4] Sensitized to rejection, the alcoholic has been said to be especially aware of the subtle, unintended cues conveyed by the doctor.

Posture and touch are additional ways we communicate, unintentionally and intentionally. Studies of postural habits have shown a wide variety of culturally patterned ways of sitting and studying. Some workers have reported a correlation between posture and certain psychologic states such as depression.[5] The logical end of proxemics or the use of space is touching.

TOUCH—WHAT IS IT?

Tactile experience is immediate, transitory, and may persist or disappear during continued contact. It is also a reciprocal experience in the sense that what a person touches also touches him, and often evokes emotional reactions of greater or lesser magnitude. Tactile experience is ordinarily limited to two persons, a means to intimacy and expression of affection or hostility and anger.[3] Once two people touch, they have eliminated the space between them, and this act usually signifies that a special type of relationship exists between them. Touching often becomes a part of an individual's style of communication. Gestures and involuntary movements unconsciously reveal a person's inner state. Psychologists call these nonverbal acts "adaptors," and they usually involve touching some part of the body with the hands. Some adaptors are unique to the individual while others are widely used and interpreted, eg, covering one's eyes with his hands may indicate concealment. Actions often do speak louder than words. Touching can help amplify or explain the meaning of what is being said, it can replace speech, it can convey inner feelings, it can be used to control the flow of conversation, and habitual gestures can be clues to one's emotional state.[6]

Touch implies that a communication is intended, but the content of the communication may not be clear. It is usually assumed that touch is an essentially positive stimulus for the recipient to the extent that it does not impose a greater level of intimacy than the recipient desires nor does it communicate a negative message.[7] Fisher and his colleagues[7] found that a casual touch of very short duration had positive consequences for the recipient, and that the effect of being touched was positive even when the touch apparently was not perceived. The response to touch was uniformly positive for women and more ambivalent for men. This corresponds with the finding that women touch and are touched by significant others more than men and that within any relationship, women report being touched more than touching.[8]

Touch among members of the same sex may be prohibited, limited to certain social situations (eg, a comforting embrace or hug with surviving relatives at a funeral), or openly encouraged. In the United States, for example, it is generally unacceptable for men to touch each other. The handshake is usually the maximal amount of touching that is permitted between American men. On the other hand, an embrace (embrazo) among Hispanic men or an exchange of kisses on the cheek by Frenchmen is usually expected in these respective cultures. Thus, the cultural background of patients and physicians will greatly influence their respective expectations about touch and the meanings ascribed to it when it occurs.

THE DOCTOR'S TOUCH

Mayerson[9] states, "Touch is a significant statement of empathy. Physical contact is a necessary maneuver to signal and establish the care-giving bond."

Schofield[10] noted that touch was often an aid in conveying thoughts. He said "in some cases a decided manner, with a hand laid firmly on the patient's arm, will enable him to assimilate suggestions otherwise inoperative." Physical contact is reassuring; when a doctor touches the patient both parties have the feeling that something is being done. Touching also means taking part; it means that matters are being taken in hand. The comfort of physical touch can be seen in how apes convey the message of reassurance; sometimes it is simply a hand touching a hand.[11]

The importance of the doctor's touch can be traced from the origins of the clinical examination. The *Nei Ching*, the oldest canon of medicine (circa 2600 BC), notes four good methods for clinical examination: the inquiry (history of complaint); inspection of the patient (color changes of skin, hair, and superficial blood vessels); auscultation (listening to the patient's heart and chest); and palpation (feeling of the pulse). The Chinese recognized the importance of pulse, which was taken in eleven places, the most important of which were the wrists. The wrist was divided into three parts, the inch, the bar, and cubit pulses—each of which represented different internal organs. A complete examination of the pulse might take up to three hours.[12] Not only did the pulse help make an anatomic diagnosis, but it detected the nature of disturbance of the Yang and Yin principles by the characteristics of the beat.

The Hindu physician Susruta noted that through the sense of touch we may know whether the skin is hot or cold, rough or smooth, thick or thin. He advocated the use of the senses in the clinical examination.

The Egyptians differed from Babylonian and Hindu physiology in their appreciation of the pulse. In the *Ebers Papyrus* (circa 1500 BC) it is said that "by feeling the pulse you feel the heart that speaks out of the vessels of every limb...."[13] The palpation of the pulse was linked with the Egyptians' conception of disease resulting from the obstruction of blood vessels. In addition, the head was palpated with the hand to detect fever. It was typical bedside manner for Egyptian physicians to touch the wound. The gesture of touching wounds, aside from hygenic considerations, suggests deeper meanings, namely those of control, reassurance, and healing.

The Greeks pursued the study of the pulse. Hippocrates added auscultation to palpation in the clinical examination. Herophilus, a follower of Hippocrates, said "to detect its exact harmony in relation to age and disease one needs to be a musician, and even a mathematician to understand the pulse."[14] However, at the same time that Hippocratic medicine was practiced, the cult of Asclepius was active. Thus, the counter-balancing of the more empirically oriented medicine of Hippocrates with that of the more mysterious, religiously oriented tradition of Asclepius and with several forms of healing in Christianity, which had roots in Babylonian and Asyrian culture. In the Roman Empire, Christians who had weak faith were regarded as evil. This is illustrated by the casting out of devils, the curative laying on of hands described in the Bible and, in England, such rituals as Touching for the King's Evil or scrofula.[12,15]

Galen combined Hippocratic methods with those of magic and religion. The combination of medicine, magic, and religion, with modifications in various cultures, led to the development of astrologic medicine, uroscopy, and pulse lore. Hence, is was not until the 17th Century, when William Harvey discovered circulation and began to bridge the gap between clinical methods of observing the cardiovascular system by demonstrating the useful potentials of measurement of bodily functions, that temperature-taking and pulse-counting were woven into the texture of medicine. Percussion and auscultation were refined with the work of Leopold Auenbrugger (percussion of the chest) in the 18th Century and Laennec (auscultation performed with the aid of stethoscope) in the early 19th Century.

The doctor's touch was also noted to be important in diagnosis in obstetrics. Cowan, in *A Bedside Manual of Physical Diagnosis* (1836), writes "to discover the motions of the child, apply the hand to the parietes and press them suddenly with a degree of succession...movements which are extremely faint or altogether imperciptible to the hand, may sometimes be very distinctly perceived by gradually pressing the cheek upon the abdomen and leaving it in contact for some time."[16]

Loomis[17] stated that there were six physical methods of diagnosis: inspection, palpation, mensuration, succussion (ear applied to surface of the chest), percussion, and auscultation. He believed percussion and auscultation were the most important of these methods, as they assisted the physician in discerning the topography of the abdomen. Laycock[18] noted that there were instruments to aid the sense of vision (the microscope) and hearing (the stethoscope), but no aid for the sense of touch. He stressed the importance of touch in the first general examination of the patient. "The patient will perhaps offer you his hand—you may derive information from this," especially the manner in which the hand is offered and the nature of the grasp.[18] Indeed, it is possible, for example, to arrive at the tentative diagnosis of hypothyroidism from an initial handshake. Such a patient's hands are likely to be cool, dry, and leathery. A world of information is imparted by a handshake, from the moist, cool hand of someone who is nervous or tense, to a host of neurologic changes (eg, hemiplegia, parkinsonism, or myasthenia gravis). The handshake, therefore, has many implications beyond touch.

The physician's eye contact and attentiveness also may physically affect the patient. Eye contact usually precedes tactile contact. The physician's touch is sensitive to form and movement; it can obtain information on temperature, resistance to palpation, force of movement or palpable vibrations; and it elicits a reaction from the patient to palpation.[19] The physician's hand may provoke pain or may manipulate parts to obtain information.

THE HEALING TOUCH

Patient's reactions to the doctor's touch or lack of it are influenced to a great extent by the expectations patients have when they seek out a doctor. Most people visit a physician when they are ill; they expect the physician to help them get well. Others visit physicians when they are troubled or worried about their real or imagined illnesses or those of relatives or friends; their expectation is that the physician will talk and listen, give advice, relieve feelings of fear or frustration or reassure them perhaps by a touch. A small number of people visit physicians periodically to check-up on their state of health; they hope the physician will give them "a clean bill of health" and a pat on the back, ie, a form of blessing, or will advise them of aspects of their health that warrant close scrutiny, ie, a form of therapy or preventive medicine.

All three groups of patients expect some form of healing or

laying on of hands by the physician. Thus, while touching has diagnostic value for the physician, touching has therapeutic value for the patient. Touching and laying on of hands, therefore, may be synonymous in the mind of the patient, while they might be seen by the physician as a religious rather than a medical action.

Historically there was a strong belief that there was healing power in the touch of a great person.[20] The Bible has many examples describing how Christ touched and healed persons with various illnesses. A touch and the sign of the cross were used in England and France by royalty to heal scrofula.[21] French and English kings were seen as having divine prerogatives and rights and thus were seen as imbued with unique powers both politically and religiously. Priests were also seen as possessing sacred powers. The fingers of the priest were important in transmitting this power to wine, water, oil, and the Host.

The touch did not always cure. Those who were not healed and complained were said to lack faith or it was said that the diagnosis was wrong. Indeed, scrofula (bovine tuberculosis) is not readily cured; it often recurs, but it can give the illusion of being cured by temporary remission. Only a certain number of people who were touched for scrofula recovered their health completely. The majority of cures took place a considerable time after the healing rite. Indeed, scrofula covered a wide variety of lesions, some of which would disappear by themselves.[15] Scrofula is still fairly common in some parts of Europe, though very rare in the United States.

The effectiveness of the laying on of hands was dependent upon several factors: that it was a private act, that its aim was unity with God and not the recovery of health, that it was not used as a last resort, and that the healer was dedicated.[22] Certainly the recipient of the laying on of hands must also be serious and well-intentioned in his desire to get well.

THE UNTOUCHABLES AND THE UNTOUCHED

Communicating by touch reaches toward the very heart of human interaction and culture. Touch is regulated by the system of ranking individuals in a particular culture. The principal forms of ranking are castes and classes. Social class may be changed, while caste is a fixed class in which rank is based on heredity. Members of the same class receive their status by birth from their parents, but they may lose or alter that status by subsequent behavior. Members of the same caste also receive their status at birth, but it remains permanently fixed regardless of their subsequent achievement.

The old Hindu social system is a classic illustration of the phenomenon of caste. The origins of the Hindu caste system seem to have been primarily ethnic stratification derived on the part of the varied peoples that have successively lived in India. The official theology of Hinduism states that there should be four castes or varna: Brahmans (priests), Kshatniyas (soldiers), Vaisyas (merchants), and Sudras (untouchables). About one fifth of India's population are the lowest caste, the untouchables. They sweep roads, clean latrines, and collect the carcasses of dead animals. The caste of each individual is unchangeable from birth and only through rebirth can he enter a higher grade. No one may marry outside his caste without loss of status. Contact with corpses is especially unclean and high-caste medical students cannot study anatomy by dissection in Indian medical schools. Mere contact with an untouchable is contaminating, and there are taboos on receiving food and drink from a low-caste person. Untouchables may not take water from the same well as high-caste persons and any food or drinking vessels belonging to a higher caste must be destroyed if used by an untouchable. Even their shadow falling on a person of higher caste is thought defiling.

Racial stratification of blacks, Hispanics, and American Indians in the United States has had certain similarities to the Indian caste system. This is evident in feelings about miscegenation, geographic avoidance, limitations on types of job and social opportunities available, and expectations of whites regarding physical intimacy between ethnic groups. While these prohibitions have diminished, they are still evident today in both overt and covert communication among different ethnic groups.

We are aware of the social and psychologic costs to the leper who is shunned by others and sentenced to live without experiencing human touch or the child with *epidermolysis bullosa hereditaria* (a loosening of the skin) who cannot be touched without further complicating this painful disorder. A recent study by Lynch[23] indicates that the lack of human contact as evidenced by loneliness can be a cause of premature death. Lynch learned that human contact no more warm and personal than a touch on a wrist for a pulse had a positive effect on a patient's heartbeat. Tactile communication is also known to have therapeutic effects, as in physical medicine and physical therapy. Touching to the patient is part of the process of getting well. Touching and being touched is an expression of caring. Remen et al.[24] have said "Human caring, sharing, feeling, accepting, touching and nourishing may all be thought of as manifestations of the feminine principle—the dimension which has been generally repressed in the modern view of professionalism." Are more patients untouched in the doctor-patient relationship? Are patients' expectations to be touched by a powerful person unfulfilled?

It is obvious that the diagnostic touch is not being abandoned in the doctor-patient relationship. Yet, with the introduction of new types of health professionals who are trained to perform clinical examinations, it is likely that the touch will not always be from a physician. While physician extenders can conduct clinical examinations competently, the patient's expectations are usually to see and be touched by *the doctor*. The doctor may not see and talk with the patient until other health professionals have conducted the necessary tests and examinations, and in some group practices and health maintenance organizations, the patient may not see the same physician each visit. Furthermore, instrumentation and medical technology have minimized touching in the doctor-patient relationship. Indeed, the current scrutiny of medical ethics and malpractice has sensitized physicians to the nature and content of the doctor-patient relationship and has perhaps encouraged some physicians to become more formal and aloof. All of these factors have led to the professionalization of the doctor-patient relationship.

Medical practice reflects our culture, its values and beliefs. Central to this culture is belief in progress through science and technology. The quality of health care depends not only on how well physicians and other health professionals perform their tasks and the reliability of the technologies they use, but also on their ability to be human. To touch and be touched is part of the process of staying well or getting well.

REFERENCES

1. L. K. Frank, Tactile communication. *Genet Psychol Monographs,* 56:209-55, 1957.
2. A. Montagu, *Touching: The Human Significance of the Skin.* New York: Columbia University Press, 1971.
3. L. K. Frank, Tactile experiences in personality development. *Genet Psychol Monographs,* 56:223-35, 1957.
4. S. Milmoe et al., The doctor's voice: posdictor of successful referral of alcoholic patients. *J Abnorm Psychol,* 72:78-84, 1967.
5. A. Mehrabian, *Nonverbal Communication.* Chicago: Aldine, 1972.
6. P. Ekman and W. V. Friesen, The repertoire of nonverbal behavior: categories, origins, usage and coding. *Semiotica, 1:*49-98, 1969.
7. J. D. Fisher, M. Rytting, and R. Heslin, Hands touching hands: affective and evaluative effects of an interpersonal touch. *Sociometry, 39:*416-21, 1976.
8. S. M. Jourard, An exploratory study of body-accessibility. *British J Soc Clin Psychol,* 5:221-31, 1966.
9. E. W. Mayerson, *Putting the Ill at Ease.* New York: Harper & Row, 1956.
10. A. T. Schofield, *The Personality of the Physician.* London: J & A Churchill, 1904.
11. M. Guido, *The Healing Hand: Man and Wound in the Ancient World.* Cambridge: Harvard University Press, 1975.
12. K. D. Keele, *The Evolution of Clinical Methods in Medicine.* Springfield: Thomas, 1963.
13. B. Ebbell, *The Papyrus Ebers.* New York: Walter DeGruyter, 1937.
14. V. Robinson, *The Story of Medicine.* New York: Tudor Press, 1931, p. 69.
15. M. Bloch, *The Royal Touch.* Translated by J. F. Anderson, London: Routledge & Kegan Paul, 1973.
16. C. Cowan, *A Bedside Manual of Physical Diagnosis.* London: Sherwood, Gilbert & Piper, 1836.
17. A. L. Loomis, *Lessons in Physical Diagnosis.* New York: Robert M. DeWitt, 1868.
18. T. Laycock, *Lectures on the Principles and Methods of Observation and Research.* Philadelphia: Blanchard & Lea, 1857.
19. J. H. Tyrer and M. J. Eadie, *The Astute Physician: How to Think in Clinical Medicine.* Amsterdam: Elsevier, 1976.
20. G. A. Duttrick (Ed.), *The Interpreter's Dictionary of the Bible.* Nashville, TN: Abingdon Press, 1962, p. 51.
21. F. L. Cross (Ed.), *The Oxford Dictionary of the Christian Church.* London: Oxford University Press, 1952.
22. L. D. Weatherhead, *Psychology, Religion and Healing.* Nashville, TN: Abingdon Press, 1951.

23. J. J. Lynch, *The Broken Heart: The Medical Consequences of Loneliness.* New York: Basic Books, 1977.

24. N. Remen, A. A. Blau, and R. Hively, *The Masculine Principle, The Feminine Principle and Humanistic Medicine.* San Francisco: Institute for the Study of Humanistic Medicine, 1975.

Chapter 6

PRE-OPERATIVE APPROACH TO PATIENTS

K. BIRKINSHAW

Established techniques of anaesthesia provide a safe and comfortable journey through the operative period for the vast majority of patients, and yet they still think of surgery as a harrowing experience. This is due to fear which has several causes.

PAIN. The amount of pain which can be expected is often unknown and may be imaged as worse than reality.

THE RISK. This is often exaggerated and patients may not have had a chance to voice their fears.

PROGNOSIS. Discussion of the outlook should be honest but tactful. The technique described below applies to non-malignant conditions. It is applicable to cancer patients but a great deal more tact and caution is required. Many patients think they have cancer when they have not.

MYSTIQUE. The old attitude was to accept without question what the doctor said or left unsaid but now this is altering. Patients are better educated and more interested than formerly. Doctors are no longer the lofty people whom patients are afraid to question. The mystique of medicine is disappearing. If a doctor is prepared to spend the time to study the technique of explanation, many patients will be delighted to respond with an improved relationship.

REASONS FOR NOT DISCUSSING MATTERS WITH THE PATIENT

LACK OF TIME. The technique to be described may take 10

Reprinted with permission from *Anaesthesia,33:*483-7, 1978.

minutes and often less. This is not long when considering the importance of an operation to the patient.

FEAR OF WORRYING THE PATIENT. Thorough explanation is like any other form of treatment accompanied by adverse side effects. Care in selection of patients and technique of delivery should minimise these fears.

THE PATIENT DOES NOT REMEMBER WHAT HE IS TOLD. This statement is true, but it may not be important. If he has been shown that the problem is understandable he does not have to remember it.

LACK OF SKILL. The correct use of language and drawing require much practice.

To allay the patient's fears pre-operatively is sufficient reason for the anaesthetist to be concerned with pre-operative explanation. The author's interest began when, as a junior, he found that many patients were facing an important event in their lives without the vaguest idea about the background to the operation. Few people would expect to face a major upheaval in any other field, be it business or legal, without thorough knowledge of the pros and cons.

This function could well be done by other doctors looking after the patient, such as the surgeon or general practitioner. One does not wish to imply that surgeons or general practitioners are lacking in their care. Medical students are taught how to obtain diagnostic information from their patients by history taking, but are not well taught about how to impart information to the patient.

The justification for the anaesthetist doing this is that it is a supplement or, in some cases, a replacement for the pre-medication. It is also true that most patients sign their consent forms without having had the explanation due to them. The part of the form to be signed by the doctor giving the explanation is often left blank. If a mishap should occur it is better to have the patient on your side beforehand rather than afterwards.

Explanation, by establishing good relations, may help prevent an action which often arises from communication failure. Our Lord says in the Gospel according to St. Matthew (Ch. 5 vs. 25-26) "Agree with thine adversary quickly whilst thou art in the way with him" (otherwise) "thou shalt not come out until thou hast paid the uttermost farthing."

It is better for a patient to be told details of his operation by a doctor than by the nurses or the patient in the next bed.

TECHNIQUE OF PRE-OPERATIVE CONSULTATION

FIRST PART. The first part of the anaesthetic consultation is conventional. A brief review of the history notes and tests is followed by any further examination necessary. It is important for the anaesthetist to sit so as not to stare down on the patient from a height, and also to give his name when the patient gives his. The object in the first part in addition to the usual purpose of a pre-anaesthetic visit is to achieve understanding with the patient, to assess his interest and intelligence and to decide whether or not to ask the question which introduces the second part.

SECOND PART. The introductory question must not be phrased so as to expect a particular answer. Examples of a suitable question are "Would you like to know more about what we are going to do tomorrow or would you rather not?", or "Are you happy with what you know about your operation or would you like me to tell you some more?"

Those likely to answer "no" are generally not asked in the first place. Unsuitable patients include children, the very old, the deaf or blind, the unintelligent, those who are abnormally anxious and those with a language barrier.

The rest usually answer "yes" happily, but if "no" then they have had the opportunity and good relations have been fostered.

To the "yes" group the technique has four stages, which may be described as, setting the scene, describing the normal structure and function, discussing the abnormality, and saying how the operation will improve symptoms. After that, one can discuss briefly pain and its relief, and then stress the importance of moving the legs and deep breathing as something that the patient can do to aid his own recovery and rapid discharge.

There are certain points in conducting this dialogue which make for clarity.

SIMPLICITY. Patients have no background knowledge so one has to start from the very beginning and go from anatomy to physiology, and then to pathology and clinical and operative surgery.

LANGUAGE. Sentences and words should be short, the active voice is used rather than the passive. One has to be didactic and not discursive.

LOGIC. The steps should be small, without missing a single one. Once the patient has lost the thread it is very laborious to pick it up again.

JARGON. If this has to be used it should be explained. The best way of doing this is to give the etymology or the story behind the word.

DRAWINGS

These are essential to the technique. They must be done quickly, simply and are in no way works of art. They can be done on any convenient surface in pen or biro. No rubbers should be used. They are best done upside down so that the patient can see them building the right way up.

Figure 6-1 sets the scene for a submucous resection, Fig. 6-2 is for any abdominal surgery on a woman and Fig. 6-3 is for a prostatectomy.

The drawings should take in a big enough area for the patient to be orientated. Then the internal structures are added while the anaesthetist tells about the normal function, the nose is described as an air conditioning plant (Fig. 6-4), the bile, as detergent for fat absorption (Fig. 6-5) and the prostate secretion as part of normal semen (Fig. 6-6).

The third set of drawings illustrate the abnormality. If we are not certain of the origin or aetiology it is better to say "We do not know why this occurs," rather than to give any theories.

In the case of the nose a fresh drawing of the part in question can be done to avoid scribbling (Fig. 6-7) and similarly with the gall bladder (Fig. 6-8). With the prostate one can show how the proper emptying of the bladder is spoilt and how the symptoms can arise (Fig. 6-9). Finally, the results of surgery are shown; the straight septum (Fig, 6-10) the gall bladder and stones removed (Fig. 6-11) and the free passage of urine down the catheter (Fig. 6-12).

QUANTITATIVE RESULTS OF A QUESTIONNAIRE

These techniques have been in use for 5 years. Recently a

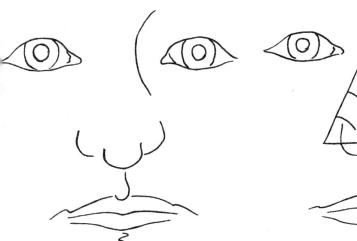

Fig. 6-1. Submucous resection.

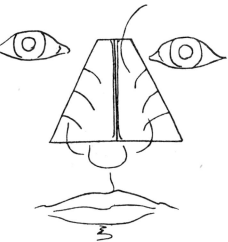

Fig. 6-4. Nasal function.

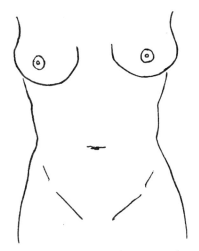

Fig. 6-2. Abdominal surgery.

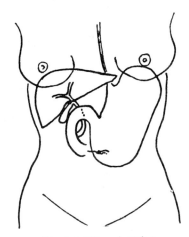

Fig. 6-5. Biliary function.

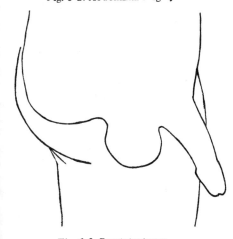

Fig. 6-3. Prostatectomy.

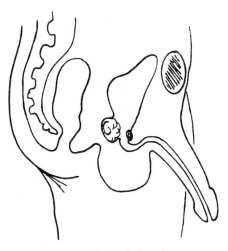

Fig. 6-6. Prostatic function.

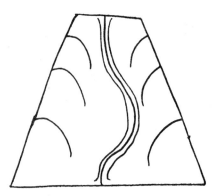

Fig. 6-7. The deflected nasal septum.

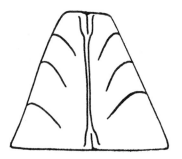

Fig. 6-10. The straight nasal septum.

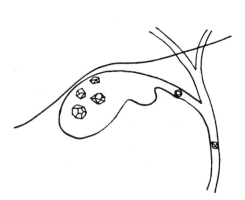

Fig. 6-8. Gallstones.

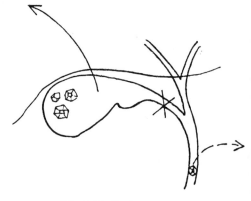

Fig. 6-11. Cholecystectomy.

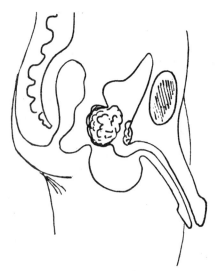

Fig. 6-9. The enlarged prostate.

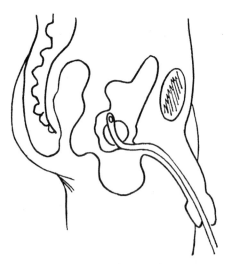

Fig. 6-12. The urinary catheter.

questionnaire has been sent to a sample of patients. The total number of questionnaires was thirty. Each patient was asked eight questions with multiple choice answers.

THE RESULTS. Most patients were relaxed during the talk, none were very nervous (26 relaxed, 4 mildly nervous, 0 very nervous). The introductory question was fair (all patients said so). The technique of language and drawing was simple enough (25 simple enough, 5 too complicated). Most patients were reassured, none were frightened (28 reassured, 2 unaffected). Two thirds had good recall and they thought recall valuable. The remainder had forgotten much of the talk but were not worried about it (21 good recall, 9 poor).

DISCUSSION

This was a pilot study only and it would be necessary to obtain bigger samples and to remove any bias due to the desire of patients to be helpful. A visual analogue scale might be valuable to grade nervousness and reassurance. Present experience, however, suggests that explanation improved patients' pre-operative morale, that the technique is about right and that if patients forget the details this does not really matter.

SUMMARY

Thorough explanation of an operation can and should be given to a large number of patients. They are selected by a non-leading question once they have been assessed, and given a logical talk with simple drawings.

A pilot questionnaire study shows that such a procedure is harmless and reassuring. It is justified as a supplement to the pre-medication but could well be done by other doctors, such as general practitioners or surgeons.

Good explanation increases patient's confidence in the surgeon, never undermines it.

Chapter 7

TECHNIQUES FOR COMMUNICATING WITH YOUR ELDERLY PATIENT

DAN BLAZER

Family physicians and internists are becoming increasingly involved in treating the physical and emotional problems of late life. Ten percent of the population of the United States is now over 65, a marked increase over the past 75 years.[1] The care of older persons is no longer confined to chronic care facilities, such as nursing homes, but is being carried out in acute care hospitals, outpatient clinics, and physicians' offices.[2] Some authors have noted that a significant percentage of the problems brought to family physicians are primarily psychologic.[3] With the increase of mental illness in late life and the chronic nature of many physical illnesses, we can assume that most of the elderly patient's medical problems will have significant psychologic components that may either be primarily responsible for the patients' symptoms, or reactions to severe and debilitating organic disorders.

Even in this sophisticated age, the patient's medical and psychosocial history remains an important diagnostic tool. The success of almost any treatment depends to a considerable extent on the adequacy of the initial history. By verbal and nonverbal communication, the patient transmits information to the clinician for use in evaluation and plans for management.

Communication is of central importance in human behavior.[4] The human personality is largely formed and shaped through communication patterns. Orderly communication between two people or among individuals within a group generally leads to adaptive behavior by each individual. However, a disordered

---

Reprinted with permission of the author from *Geriatrics, 33*:79-84, 1978.

96

communication pattern can lead to disordered or maladaptive behavior. For example, misunderstandings between physician and patient may lead to behavior patterns that are nontherapeutic for the patient and frustrating for the physician. In fact, this country's malpractice crisis probably results more from poor communication between physicians and patients than from incompetent medical care. If psychologic factors are involved in most illnesses managed by the family practitioner and internist, then communication is necessary for treatment and evaluation. The technique is principally used in psychotherapy to produce beneficial behavior change.[5] The modern physician is intervening earlier, and is taking a more active role in the diagnosis and management of diseases of the elderly. Communication between the physician and the older patient plays a major role in the physician's ability to work effectively with the elderly. Factors that aid communication, and guidelines to effective communication, between elderly patient and the physician will be discussed in this article.

FACTORS INFLUENCING COMMUNICATION WITH THE ELDERLY

In every human interaction, each participant makes a contribution that will influence the outcome. Both the patient and the physician must be considered as individuals before interaction can be understood properly. Factors influencing each may be assets or barriers to effective communication.

Patient Factors

ANXIETY. Many elderly individuals may function continually at a high level of anxiety. Thus, the increased stress of a new situation may lead to intense arousal, impairing the elderly person's ability to communicate effectively.[6] Every physician realizes that a visit to the doctor is often a stressful experience. Fear, shame, anxiety, and a host of other feelings may play an important role in the communication process in the physician's office.

SENSORY DEPRIVATION.[7] Hearing loss is a widespread problem among the elderly. It affects men more than women and occurs in some 30% of all older people. Hearing loss is potentially the most difficult sensory loss for the elderly patient. Although 80% of the elderly have fair to adequate vision, some visual problems may occur. For example, poor orientation, a decreasing ability to read, and an occasional frightening visual impression may complicate communication in the physician's office.

CAUTIOUSNESS. Older persons tend to make few errors of commission but are likely to make errors of omission.[8] When the physician takes a history, he or she must be aware that older people may omit important aspects of their illnesses. Older people also take longer to respond to inquiries. The physician who rushes through the history-taking may overlook valuable information.

UNREALISTIC VIEWS OF THE PHYSICIAN. The elderly patient may develop an unrealistic perception of the physician based on previous experiences (the process that psychiatrists call transference). The elderly person is likely to view the physician as a parent (leading to a marked dependence on the patient's part), or as a child (leading to instruction-giving, or inquiries about the physician's health and behavior). A positive transference can be of benefit in the management of the patient if handled properly.

PERSISTENT THEMES. The elderly patient may concentrate on particular themes in communicating with the physician. The more common themes include:

Somatic concern: Patients may spend much time complaining of ailments or recounting detailed histories of bodily functions. At a time when friends and loved ones have died and sensory input is decreased, the body, in many ways, keeps the patient company. It is therefore quite usual for the elderly patient to be somatically oriented.[9]

Loss reactions: The elderly patient may spend considerable time discussing the many losses experienced in late life. These include loss of friends and loved ones, loss of physical functioning, loss of employment and previous activities, and loss of self-esteem.

Life review:[10] There is a tendency in the elderly to reflect and reminisce. This is a normal process brought about by disillusion and the realization that death is approaching.

Fear of losing control:[11] Many elderly patients agonize over the loss of physical and mental functions, including physical strength, bowel and bladder control, motor functions, and, especially, the ability to regulate one's thoughts and emotions. One of the greatest fears of late life is the fear of "going crazy."

Death: The elderly are not, as a rule, obsessed with approaching death, but it nevertheless is a frequent topic of conversation. The major fear is of being alone at the end of life. The physician must remember the importance of continued relationships for the elderly person.

Physician Factors

ATTITUDES TOWARD THE ELDERLY. It is quite common to find fears of aging and death among members of our youth-oriented society.[12] The recognition of such fears and of the physician's personal feelings about these issues is of utmost importance in establishing effective communication with the elderly.

LACK OF UNDERSTANDING. The physician must attempt to separate myths about aging from reality. For example, the labeling and stereotyping of the elderly may be a significant barrier to communication. The elderly are especially sensitive to being labeled "senile," "mentally ill," or "hypochondriac." The physician should try to empathize with the elderly patient. Putting yourself in the other person's shoes is an ability not easily taught by textbooks and can only be learned through personal experiences.

TECHNIQUES OF EFFECTIVE COMMUNICATION

APPROACH THE ELDERLY PATIENT WITH RESPECT. The physician should knock before entering the examining room and try to approach the patient from the front. Greet the patient by surname (Mr. Smith, Mrs. Ross) rather than by given name (Johnny, Mary), unless he or she wishes to be addressed by a given name.

POSITION YOURSELF NEAR THE OLDER PATIENT. The physician should place himself or herself near enough to be able to reach out and touch the patient if desired. The most comfortable arrangement of chairs for both parties is at a 45-degree angle to each other. If possible, chairs should be of the same height and the physician should not stand or walk during the interview.

SPEAK CLEARLY AND SLOWLY. The elderly patient may have a hearing problem or may not understand a physician's accent. Clarity of speech and the use of simple sentences is most effective in communicating with an elderly patient, especially for those who have a hearing loss or organic brain disease.

The staff of the OARS Clinic at the Center for the Study of Aging at Duke University found that telephone interviews with older patients are effective for gathering initial information and for follow-up. The telephone enables the patient to take advantage of preserved bone conduction in mild to moderate hearing loss.

INQUIRE ACTIVELY AND SYSTEMATICALLY INTO THE PROBLEMS PRESENTED. The physician should inquire into common physical symptoms of late life (such as visual and auditory defects, falls, and weight loss) and typical psychosocial problems (death of a loved one, change in living arrangements, recent retirement, financial setbacks, feelings of decreased self-esteem, hopelessness, and anxiety).

PACE THE INTERVIEW. The elderly patient must be given enough time to respond to the physician's questions. The elderly are not, as a rule, uncomfortable with silences, which give them an opportunity to formulate answers to questions, and to elaborate on certain points. A slow and relaxed pace in the interview will do much to decrease anxiety.

PAY ATTENTION TO NONVERBAL COMMUNICATION. The physician should be alert for changes in facial expressions, gestures, postures, and touch as auxiliary methods of communication in the elderly. These nonverbal signs can provide considerable information about conditions such as depression or anxiety.

Touch may also be an effective way to relax and make contact with the elderly patient. As a rule, the elderly are less inhibited about physical touch. Holding the patient's hand or resting your hand on his arm may be very reassuring.

BE REALISTIC BUT HOPEFUL. Physicians who work with the elderly often deny the problems of late life. But neither the patient nor the physician believes phrases like "You'll live to be a hundred," or "It's nothing to worry about," and the physician should avoid using them, He should never abandon all hope for a particular patient, but should work in the here and now, avoiding unrealistic expectations. Two or three pain-free days may be most rewarding to the patient dying of cancer, a fact too often overlooked by the frustration physician.

CONTINUE THE RELATIONSHIP WITH THE ELDERLY PATIENT. The internist and family physician should avoid, as much as possible, permanent transfer and termination of care of elderly patients. A visit to the physician's office is often a social event in the elderly patient's life. The physician and other health care personnel become important individuals to the elderly. Getting "well" may mean the loss of contact with treasured associates.

Many clinicians working with the elderly have found that regular but infrequent checkups are quite reassuring for elderly patients. Most of them will not abuse such an open door policy.

REFERENCES

1. H. B. Brotman, Who are the aging? In E. W. Busse and E. Pfeiffer (Eds.), *Mental Illness in Later Life*. Washington, D.C.: American Psychological Association, 1973.
2. E. Pfeiffer, Interacting with older people. In Busse and Pfeiffer, *op. cit.*
3. M. Shepherd, General practice and mental illness and the British National Health Service. *Pub Health, 64*:230-33, 1974.
4. E. Pfeiffer, Communication: general and theoretical considerations, In F. R. Hine and E. Pfeiffer (Eds.), *Behavioral Science: A Selected View*. Boston: Little, Brown, 1972.
5. J. Ruesch, Therapeutic communication.
6. C. Eisdorfer, Arousal and performance: experiments in verbal learning and a tentative theory. In G. A. Falland (Ed.), *Human Aging and Behavior*. New York: Academic Press, 1968.
7. R. N. Butler and M. I. Lewis, *Aging and Mental Health*. St. Louis: C. V. Mosby, 1973.
8. J. Botwink, Cautiousness in advanced age. *J Gerontol, 21*:347, 1966.
9. A. Verwoerdt, *Clinical Geropsychiatry*. Baltimore: Williams &Wilkins, 1976.
10. R. N. Butler, The life reviewer: an interpretation of reminiscence in the aged. *Psychiatry, 26*:65, 1963.
11. J. J. Strain and S. Grossman, *Psychosocial Care of the Medically Ill*. New York: Appleton-Century-Crofts, 1975.
12. J. H. Bunzel, Recognition, relevance and the de-activation of gerontophobia. *J Am Geriatr Soc, 21*:77-80, 1973.

Chapter 8

COMMUNICATING WITH THE
HARD-OF-HEARING

CHRISTINE MCNAMEE

Perhaps the most distinctively human of all handicaps is impairment of the capacity to comprehend language. Breakdown in an individual's ability to communicate with others through the use of language has many effects. It is the most clearly identifiable factor complicating and deepening maladjustment in the mentally and emotionally disturbed. It often accompanies the normal aging process.

Studies have shown that sensory loss ranks second as a cause of low morale among the elderly.[1] Some theorists believe that delusions of persecution as well as hallucinations in the elderly stem directly from sensory deprivation. If you cannot hear, it is difficult to understand with any accuracy what is going on.

One out of every four people over the age of 65 is affected to some degree by hearing loss. It may be caused by a decrease in overall sensitivity to sound, or by selective loss of hearing for higher pitches. The former is due to mechanical problems caused by ossification of the articulating bones of the inner ear, and can be corrected by surgery, use of a hearing aid, or both. The latter is due to neurological changes, and is not reversible.

Burnside suggests an effective exercise for trying to understand the handicap brought about by hearing loss.[2] Adjust the car radio volume to slightly less than normal (stimulating overall loss of sensitivity). Then, turn the tone adjustment to full bass (simulating selective loss of high pitches. Although you will still be able

Reproduced with permission from *The Canadian Nurse*, Volume 74 Number 3, 1978, pp.27-29.

to hear, you will probably have to strain in order to understand what is being said.

Although certain hearing problems can be improved through the use of a hearing aid, this is not true of all of them. The cause of hearing loss must be determined by a certified hearing specialist, and if a prosthesis is indicated, it should be prescribed and filled by this specialist, an individual who is not in the business of selling aids. Hundreds of elderly people are bilked by unscrupulous door-to-door peddlers who sell them hearing aids that are useless for their type of hearing loss. Burnside cites an example of one elderly woman who died leaving 36 hearing aids in her drawer.[3]

HEARING LOSS—WHAT IT MEANS

In addition to a fundamental knowledge of anatomy, physiology, neurology, and the pathology of hearing, we as nurses need to have a basic understanding of what hearing loss means to the individual in order to communicate effectively with him. In order to understand, we must look at the physiological, psychological and sociological effects of hearing loss.

Physiological effects may include dizziness, poor balance, or both, if there is middle ear involvement. The hard-of-hearing may suffer from fatigue because they have to concentrate harder in order to hear. Head noises are common, and these disturb rest and may result in tension and irritability. Finally, adaptive posturing such as squinting, grimacing, frowning and head tilting can give the person who is hard of hearing a rather odd appearance, so that people may respond to him in a negative way.

To recognize the psychological effects of hearing loss, we need only think for a moment. Hearing is something we all tend to take for granted and its loss is frightening and demoralizing. Hesitancy and fear of involvement in social activities are very common among the hard-of-hearing. The individual may feel that he is incapable of participating; he may fear rejection. Sensory deprivation may also result in emotional flatness, passivity, dependency and boredom. Often he will have impaired interpersonal relationships, so that his needs for affection and a sense of belonging are not fulfilled.

Someone who is hard-of-hearing may develop rigid defenses,

so that he will exhibit what seems to be an unreasonable fear of physical or psychological intrusion. It is also very easy for him to imagine that others are talking about him, almost to the point of a mild paranoia.

Our society places a high value on wholeness and functionality. For this reason deafness can result in social isolation; the individual who is hard-of-hearing may be forced into withdrawal. He may be incorrectly labelled apathetic, goalless, uninvolved, unmotivated, senile, or even schizoid. He may suffer from loss of status because it is easier to exclude him from activities and decision-making as he is an inconvenience. His self-respect may suffer when people regard him as simple because of his lack of comprehension.

SENSITIVE COMMUNICATION

Loss of hearing can have profound effects on an individual. If we understand these effects, we can also see how important it is to maintain effective communication with those who are hard-of-hearing. Awareness of the following points may help the quality of communication and the relationship that develops between the nurse and the patient who is hard-of-hearing.

1. *The responsibility for understanding conversation does not rest entirely with the person who is hard-of-hearing.* In the hospital situation, it is partly the nurse's responsibility. This has important implications with regard to safety consideration, especially in such matters as preoperative instruction, where the patient's safety depends on his comprehension. In these cases, return demonstrations and verbal feedback can serve as checks of comprehension.

2. *Reassurance is very important for the patient since he may misinterpret sounds or misunderstand communications.* Body language, always of great importance, assumes even greater significance in any interaction with the hard-of-hearing. This individual has learned to rely on his eyes to help him hear, much as someone who is blind depends on heightened auditory acuity. The nurse's ability to communicate warmth and understanding through body language is especially important in establishing a trusting relationship with the patient.

3. *Get the patient's attention before you speak, by calling his*

name or gently touching his arm. Then he will be ready to concentrate on your words. He may not have heard your approach, especially in a hospital setting, where nurses wear soft-soled shoes.

4. *Remember that medications may affect his ability to pay attention.*

5. *Most hearing problems are not improved by loudness—it doesn't help to shout at someone wearing a hearing aid.* Shouting can distress the patient unnecessarily because it means loss of privacy. It may also offend the sensibilities of nearby patients, particularly if what you are shouting is of a personal nature. It may also disturb their rest.

6. *Speak clearly, and not too quickly.*

7. *Face the person directly, and keep your hands away from your mouth when you're talking.* Many of those who are hard of hearing depend on lip-reading to augment their hearing capacity. For this reason, it is also wise to consider lighting when conversing with such a patient: make sure it is sufficient to allow him to see your lip movements clearly.

Attempts at conversing with the patient when his back is turned to you, as during back care or bedmaking, will probably result in anxiety and frustration for him. He may not feel free to mention his discomfort to you, because he recognizes that you are trying to be pleasant.

8. *Know which side is affected.* Not all patients have bilateral hearing loss; even if they do, the degree of hearing loss may differ. If this is the case, attempts to converse with the patient when his good ear is turned into the pillow will likely be unsatisfactory. Always stand on the side of the bed corresponding to his good ear, to take advantage of the unique funnel-like anatomy of the outer ear.

9. *A foreign accent is a problem for the hearing impaired, so if you have an accent, be prepared to use a pen and paper.* Remember too that for foreign born patients for whom English is a second language, we are the ones who are difficult to understand.

10. *When you are asked to repeat a sentence a couple of times, find a different way of saying the same thing,* rather than repeating your original words over and over. It may be a particular syllable or tone that is causing the difficulty.

11. *Never use the patient's deafness as an excuse to talk over him to another nurse, doctor or visitors.* Remember the tendency of the hard-of-hearing to imagine that others are talking about him. And think of how frustrating it is to be excluded in this way.

12. *Background noises such as traffic sounds, television, and radios, make listening and hearing more difficult.*

13. *Gestures can be very useful if they enhance what you have to say.* Aimless gestures only serve to distract the patient.

14. *Accusations that the hard-of-hearing person "Hears only what he wants" are unjust.* In order to pick up information, he must concentrate harder and he tires easily. So, in actuality, he does hear "only what he can." When he is tired or distracted or ill, he is less able to hear and to understand. His ability to hear changes with each situation and with each speaker.

15. *Impatience with his listening behavior will not help,* but will only cause him to become tense and hear less. This applies also if the patient is made to feel that you are rushed. The more relaxed and accepted the hard-of-hearing person feels, the better he can communicate.

You will notice that the points I have mentioned imply sensitivity. If you understand the physiological, psychological and sociological effects of hearing loss, and recognize the hearing impaired individual as an individual with communication needs, you will be sensitive. Such sensitivity can only contribute to a mutually satisfying nurse-client relationship.

REFERENCES

1. Margaret Clark, *Culture and Aging: An Anthropological Study of Older Americans.* Springfield, Thomas, 1967.
2. Irene M. Burnside, *Nursing and the Aged.* New York: McGraw-Hill, 1976.
3. *Ibid.*

Chapter 9

INTERVIEW TECHNIQUES FOR DIAGNOSING ALCOHOLISM

Jon R. Weinberg

A lcoholism has been described as the nation's leading health problem, affecting an estimated 5 percent of American adults. At least one out of 10 men who drink at all is an alcoholic. Because most people develop the early and middle stages of the illness during their 20s or 30s, family physicians have an opportunity, if not a fundamental obligation, to establish routine screening procedures for all their adult patients. Treating the late-stage complications of this normally progressive disorder is a relatively unrewarding task. Thus, the physician makes an enormous contribution by diagnosing and helping alcoholics in the earlier stages, when most of them are capable of complete remission or marked improvement.

THE PHYSICIAN'S ATTITUDE

There are two related issues to be considered before an interview procedure is established: the physician's attitude toward drinking and the definition of alcoholism. To be effective in discussing alcohol use with his patients, the physician must first scrutinize his own feelings on the matter.

Two attitudinal problems are especially common. One is the historic view of alcoholism as a moral problem, which most people still carry deep inside them. Such feelings may lead to a subtle communication of hostility or condemnation which will block the success of the interview. The other problem is the

Reprinted with permission from the March 1974 issue of *American Family Physician*, published by the American Academy of Family Physicians.

tendency to judge the deviance of the patient's drinking pattern by comparison with the physician's habits. Physicians who drink very little or not at all may exaggerate the patient's drinking problems, while those physicians with heavier intakes may become highly reluctant to identify as alcoholic anyone who apparently drinks less.

These difficulties may be remedied by careful review and acceptance of the definition of alcoholism given in the AMA *Manual on Alcoholism.* Alcoholism is described as a chronic illness with certain identifiable characteristics, including continuing impairment of social, emotional, occupational and/or physical functioning as a direct result of alcohol use. This definition has important implications for the attitudinal problems mentioned before. First, because alcoholism qualifies as an illness, it is not appropriately viewed as a moral problem. Second, because the results of drinking, not the quantities consumed, are the paramount issue in diagnosis, there is no need for contrasting the physician's intake with that of the patient.

The basic question is this: is drinking often followed by behavior which the individual or, more commonly, others close to him find objectionable, which recurs regardless of his intentions and which would not occur if he did not drink? An affirmative answer that is diagnostic of alcoholism can be illustrated by a simple but classic example: Almost every time a couple goes to a social gathering, the man—normally pleasant— becomes intoxicated, berates his wife in front of the group and feels terrible when reminded of his behavior the next day. He sincerely tries not to do this again—but despite his best efforts the whole scenario is repeatedly reenacted.

THE DRINKING HISTORY: GROSS SCREENING

As a routine segment of the medical history, gross screening for alcohol problems usually requires only a minute or two. Variations from normal are more readily apparent if three or four standardized questions are consistently used. The specific content of these questions is not particularly critical; what requires minute attention is the style and quality of the response. Most patients can be placed into three general categories, according to these initial responses.

The first group, representing the great majority of patients in the average practice, comprises those who answer the questions as matter-of-factly as they are asked. These patients are in no way threatened by the issue and show no evidence of any difficulties with alcohol. For this group, alcoholism may be ruled out with a reasonable degree of safety unless there are independent indications, such as suspicious physical findings or a spouse's report.

Patients in the second group also give reasonable straightforward responses but express concern about their drinking and, with encouragement, freely describe the difficulties causing the concern. This group is composed of probable early stage alcoholics, symptomatic drinkers and other high-risk individuals (plus an occasional false-positive respondent who, because of mistaken information, may be needlessly concerned about a normal drinking pattern). The physician will find most of these people quite gratifying to work with, since they often respond as cooperatively as a patient with any other developing health problem.

In these cases, the physician generally will want to discuss with the patient and the spouse the symptoms and progressive nature of alcoholism, the desirability of abstaining from alcohol and, if drinking is to continue, the necessity of following a pattern of extreme moderation if serious problems are to be avoided. The patient's drinking behavior would from then on be closely monitored for any evidence of progression toward overt alcoholism. In many instances, stress factors conducive to drinking will also require close attention.

The third group is characterized by responses which appear to have the goal of persuading the physician that there is no alcohol problem, that the patient is simply another social drinker. This group consists of the probable middle stage alcoholics, whose responses reflect the elaborate system of alibis and denial that is generated to shield the person from perceiving reality. For the purpose of gross diagnostic screening, this is the group which the physician must be most carefully attuned to, so that a more definitive diagnostic assessment may follow.

Examples of suitable questions for the gross screening interview, with typical responses from the three groups described, are given in Table IX-1. The physician should introduce the subject of drinking when he is well into the overall medical history, so

TABLE IX-1
SAMPLE GROSS SCREENING QUESTIONS AND TYPICAL RESPONSES OF THREE GROUPS

Question	Nonalcoholic	Early-stage alcoholic	Middle-stage alcoholic
Has anyone ever said that drinking might be causing a problem for you?	No.	Not directly—but I've been wondering about it myself.	I can quit any time I want to—I can handle it myself.
Has your wife (husband) ever complained about your drinking?	I don't recall her ever saying anything about it.	She does get upset with me when I drink too much.	She's a nut when it comes to drinking—besides, she gripes about everything.
How much do you drink on the average?	Let's see, I suppose it would average out to around three drinks a day.	Very little during the week but I kind of let loose on weekends.	I never drink more than two and I never drink before noon.
Have you ever had to consider cutting down on your drinking?	No, except when I'm trying to lose weight.	It has crossed my mind that I'd be better off if I did.	There's no problem for me—I can take it or leave it.

that a base line of response style will have been established. Subtle deviations in patient response, such as inappropriate smiling, an undercurrent of hostility or unnecessarily discursive answers, will then be more apparent. One suggested method of opening the topic is by saying, "Now I'd like to learn a bit about your use of alcoholic beverages. Do you drink at all?"

THE DRINKING HISTORY: DETAILED INTERVIEW

After the brief gross screening, patients in whom alcoholism cannot be tentatively ruled out require a more detailed assessment. Even patients whose initial responses indicate probable middle-stage alcoholism must be given a thorough interview so that sufficient information will be available to use in the next, or pretreatment, phase. The detailed interview may take from five to 20 minutes when done skillfully.

Nonjudgmental Acceptance

The primary difference between diagnostic interviewing of suspected alcoholics and most other medical history taking is in the denial and defensiveness which are so characteristic in the former. It is critically important that the physician fully accept that the denial system is an intrinsic component of the illness. Thus, the extra difficulty and effort required to elicit pertinent information should not arouse hostility or otherwise interfere with communicating an atmosphere of nonjudgmental acceptance.

It may be helpful to keep in mind the similarity between an alcoholic and a paranoid schizophrenic in terms of manifesting a system of delusions. Few physicians would get angry at a patient who believed that people on the street constantly talked abut him or that the radio was sending him secret messages. It is no more sensible to be angry at the alcoholic who insists he drinks only one or two beers or who says he beats his wife when he drinks only because she so richly deserves it.

Directness

It is helpful to ask highly specific, factual questions which are difficult to answer evasively or vaguely. The interviewer interested in obtaining maximum diagnostic information in minimum time will want to use the following criterion in selecting a question: is the response likely to help rule in or out a diagnosis of alcoholism? Therefore, questions should lead to factual data reflecting possible adverse behavioral consequences of drinking. Since physicians seem entirely comfortable with direct questions in more traditional medical areas (such as queries about bowel function), it is likely that the reason for more oblique approaches on the drinking issue is anxiety over the possibility of hostility from the patient, or at least embarrassment.

Examples of vague or oblique questions which would not generally be helpful are: "How do you get along with your wife?," "How are things going at work?" and "How do you feel when you drink?" Examples of specific questions which are nevertheless irrelevant to diagnosis would be: "What do you drink—martinis, vodka, bourbon, scotch?" and "Do you generally like a drink before dinner?" Illustrations of direct, relevant questions are found in Table IX-2.

Persistence

A principle of particular importance, which is closely related to directness, is that of persistence. The alcoholic's denial system will often lead him to answer specific, factual questions in a way that does not yield specific, factual information. Sometimes he will evade the question entirely by, for example, telling an irrelevant anecdote about himself or someone else ("Now my Uncle Fred *really* drinks") or suddenly introducing a titillating new organic symptom ("Did I tell you about my heart attacks?"). In other cases, he may gloss over the issue with a vague or generalized response ("I suppose that could have happened").

Sometimes he will simply try to sidestep the specific issue by repeating his assurances that he can handle liquor, can quit drinking any time and has no alcohol problem. If the question is not clearly answered, the physician's best strategy is to repeat the question exactly, just as if he had not heard the patient's first response. If the answer is still unsatisfactory, he should say in a friendly way, "Now let me ask that question once again," and then do so. Not only will the patient probably then answer it but he will usually get the message that his evasive tactics will not

TABLE IX-2
EXAMPLES OF DIAGNOSTIC INTERVIEW QUESTIONS BY CONTENT AREA

NOTE: Questions underlined should be asked only if affirmative answers have been given to the questions immediately preceding them.

FAMILY LIFE:	Have you had any real physical battles with your wife (husband)? <u>Did that happen only when you were drinking?</u>
	Has your wife (husband) ever threatened divorce or even gone to a lawyer? <u>Was drinking one of the things she (he) said was a problem?</u>
	Have your teenagers ever said, or even implied, that they disapproved of your drinking? <u>What do they say they don't like about it?</u>
	Have any of your relatives suggested it might be better if you drank less or quit? <u>What exactly don't they like about your behavior when you drink?</u>
SOCIAL LIFE:	Has any friend or neighbor ever made any comment about your drinking? <u>What exactly did they say?</u>
	Does it seem as though your wife doesn't want to go out with you as much as she used to? <u>Is it possible that this change has something to do with drinking?</u>
OCCUPATIONAL FUNCTIONING:	Have you been late to work or missed any work recently? <u>Was this because of a "morning-after"?</u>
	Have you ever been laid off or let go from a job? <u>Was drinking involved in any way?</u>
LEGAL INVOLVEMENT:	Have you ever been arrested, including traffic charges? <u>Would you tell me what the charge was in each case?</u>
	Did the disorderly conduct (shoplifting, etc.) charge occur when you were drinking? <u>Do you ever get into trouble like that when you're not drinking?</u>

succeed. Consequently, his answers will often become more direct.

Never Discuss Alibis

When the patient finally reveals specific data documenting adverse consequences of drinking, he will then typically try to explain away the evidence with elaborate stories intending to show that factors other than drinking were responsible. For example, he may say, "You'd drink too if you were married to my wife" or "That boss just used drinking as an excuse to fire me—he knew I was smarter than he was." In these cases, the physician should remember an important diagnostic interview principle: never discuss alibis.

If the alibi is reasonably brief, it is best to wait until the patient finishes a sentence and then immediately go on to the next question. If the patient begins to ramble on, the physician should interrupt him in midsentence if necessary, to ask the next question. If he still persists in his story, the physician should say in a firm but friendly way, "We can come back to that later on — but now I want to ask you about something else," and then do so. If this principle is not observed, much time will be wasted and the physician will either have to reinforce the alibi or argue with the patient.

Titrate Hostility

The whole issue of drinking is extremely threatening to the alcoholic. Even the most accepting and friendly interviewer will at times observe that a patient, by verbal or nonverbal signs, is showing acute discomfort, most often in the form of anger. The principle to keep in mind is: titrate hostility.

The ultimate objective of the physician-patient relationship is not diagnosis but helpful treatment. For this reason, it is imperative to keep the probability high that the patient will return; otherwise, the energy spent on diagnosis will probably be wasted. This requires constant monitoring of the patient's level of hostility. Whenever the physician feels that he is losing rapport to the extent that the patient may end the interview or the relationship, it is advisable to shift to a subject that is not at all threatening, such as an organic issue. The drinking history may then be completed after the patient has calmed down, if time permits, or it may be put aside to approach in a subsequent interview.

In some cases, if the physician is particularly skillful at psychiatric interviewing or has known the patient for a long time, he may wish to risk a different strategy. This approach involves dealing directly with the hostility, perhaps beginning with a comment such as, "It seems to me that these questions about drinking are getting you a bit riled up." Such an approach should be attempted only if the physician feels well equipped to deal with the barrage of defensive tactics likely to ensue.

Some Interview Issues

It is not uncommon for an alcoholic to ask during the drinking history, "You don't think I'm an alcoholic, do you?" The physician should carefully refrain from responding with a yes or no to this question, since either answer will prove harmful at this point. A suggested response is, "Right now I'm trying to learn if drinking might be causing some problems in your life." Because of the stigma attached to alcoholism, emotional reactions to the word are so strong that the physician should avoid using it throughout the diagnostic phase. Later on it can be introduced with sufficient explanation to soften the patient's reaction.

A second issue is the problem of qualified answers. When direct, relevant questions are asked, the patient may give a response that is superficially negative but nevertheless is subtly qualified. Examples of such responses are: "Not as a rule"; "I wouldn't say so"; "No more than anyone else"; "Not really"; "Nothing recently"; "Practically never"; "I don't think so"; "Nothing worth mentioning"; "Probably not."

It is of critical importance that the physician be on the alert for such qualified denials, so that with his next question he can try to elicit the reason behind the qualification. For example, a response of "I wouldn't say so" may be followed by "Who would say so?", or "Practically never" by "When does it happen?" Often such exploration of qualified responses will reveal the most pertinent diagnostic information, which would otherwise be overlooked.

A third issue is the termination of the interview. The patient is likely to be, at the very least, unhappy about the intensive investigation of his drinking-related problems. Since the physician's goal is to continue the relationship, it is unwise to have the patient leave the interview with the drinking history as a central focus. It is advisable to reserve the last few minutes of the interview for discussion of the presenting complaint or other less threatening material, with no mention of drinking, even if there is a connection with alcohol use, such as gastritis or insomnia. In some cases, this may mean waiting for the next visit to complete the drinking history. Once the physician is reasonably confident he is dealing with alcoholism, the quality of the doctor-patient relationship becomes of paramount importance in the success of subsequent treatment strategies—and patience is the byword. Naturally the physician must be prepared to offer a medical reason to support a further appointment. Occasionally the reason must be partially fabricated, such as discussing the results of a minor laboratory procedure.

The only exception to the previous discussion of termination would be the rare case when the patient makes it clear, or the physician has a very strong feeling, that no further appointments will materialize. In such a situation, the physician will best fulfill his presponsibility by confronting the patient with his diagnostic impression. Even though the patient may be angry as he leaves, the truth has been stated. That tiny chip in the denial system may someday make another professional's job a bit easier or otherwise help the patient eventually face reality.

CONTENT AREAS

Since the diagnostic interview is intended to elicit facts about adverse behavior due to drinking, questions should be designed to cover the key areas in the patient's life. Most important is family life, followed by social life, occupational functioning, legal involvement and physical health. This sequence also represents the most typical chronology of problems as they develop during the progression of the patient's illness (See Table IX-2).

Family Life

Impairment of family life is most often represented by a deteriorating marital relationship. In the earlier years, arguments while drinking or quarrels about the "night before" are most frequent and some physical abusiveness is quite common. The couple's sexual relations and social life usually decrease as a result of their unpleasant associations with drinking. Later the mate may threaten or actually initiate separation or divorce. While a few mates (wives, generally) become sullenly tolerant of the alcoholic's behavior after a number of years, most continue to voice their dissatisfaction. The physician should attempt to determine the degree of dissatisfaction, the nature of the drinking behavior which produced it and any evidence suggesting that the mate will end the relationship. If the patient has a history of divorce, the possible role of drinking problems in the previous marriage(s) should be investigated.

It is often valuable to include questions about relationship with any preadolescent or older children. They tend to draw away from the alcoholic because of his unpredictable extremes of behavior and often they avoid bringing friends home because of the risk of embarrassment. (For example, when they walked in, mom may be passed out on the couch; dad might be drunk and obnoxious).

With unmarried patients, the physician may ask about concern by parents, siblings, other relatives, roommates or steady dates. For example, a serious relationship may have been broken off before marriage because of drinking or an older sister or brother may have tried to talk to the patient about his toxic behavior.

Social Life

While many alcoholics, especially women, confine most of their drinking to their own homes, it is more common for them to seek social environments where drinking is the norm, as in taverns, bars or private clubs. As a person's drinking behavior shifts from a social to an alcoholic pattern, he naturally seeks drinking companions with whom he feels comfortable, that is, those who do not make his own behavior appear deviant. As a result, he spends much less time with old friends and cultivates a new group whose primary bond is drinking. The physician should ask about such social changes over the years, as well as any direct comments about the patient's drinking by old friends or neighbors.

As mentioned before, drinking problems often result in less frequent socializing by the couple. The patient's wife may feel embarrassment with their old friends and resentment or boredom with the heavy-drinking new crowd. This may lead the patient to describe his wife as a "party poop." The key factor to assess here is whether the wife's resistance reflects a change in her social interest produced primarily by the husband's drinking behavior.

Occupational Functioning

The physician may find several clues to impaired job performance which could be related to alcohol use. These include: frequent job changes, loss of job, periods of unemployment, failure to advance within an organization, absences from work (especially on Mondays), tardiness, inefficiency and moving toward jobs where there is freedom to drink unobserved (house painter, real estate salesman, traveling salesman) or which are difficult to be fired from (civil service). Since employment problems usually develop only late in the drinking career, if ever, many alcoholics have an excellent job record at the time of the physicians assessment. Nevertheless, impaired occupational functioning is an important sign.

Patients who are not in regular paid employment, such as housewives, students and those on retirement or disability income may be questioned to determine whether performance of whatever daily tasks they have is being impaired by drinking.

Legal Involvement

It is useful to learn the charges in all arrests the patient has ever had as an adult (if any) and whether drinking was a factor in any of them. The most typical relevant legal offense uncovered, especially in higher income groups, is driving while intoxicated. A record of two or more such charges is virtually presumptive of alcoholism. Sometimes the conviction is for a lesser charge or is even dismissed, so it is more useful to ask about the arrest. A pattern of frequent auto accidents may also prove relevant.

Other than driving, such offenses as assault, disorderly conduct, resisting arrest and most petty crimes against property are often alcohol related; these occur more frequently in lower income groups. Any arrests for public drunkenness, still considered a crime in most states, are of obvious significance.

Physical Health

While the family physician has intimate knowledge of the patient's current physical status, certain issues may require inquiry. For example, medical care which antedated the current physician's involvement should be looked into. Did any previous physician suggest that drinking be curtailed? Were any injuries or illnesses related to drinking? Have withdrawal symptoms been experienced?

It should also occur to the physician to examine more closely the cause of any accidents that involved cigarette burns, falling down or bumping into things (for example, a housewife's bruised shins). Other observations may be revealing: An odor of alcohol during an office visit is extremely suggestive, as are late-night phone calls which are not fully coherent. An unusual number of cancelled or missed appointments is also suspicious.

INFORMATION FROM OTHERS

Obtaining information from intimates of the suspected alcoholic is the most efficient method of making a correct diagnosis. Usually an objective history can be elicited because there is no denial system to contend with. The spouse is the most likely person from whom to seek a history. If the spouse is also the physician's patient, there is an excellent chance that he or she has already made some spontaneous comments or complaints ("He's so nice when he's sober but..."). Thus, the physician will probably find it easy to obtain a more detailed history from the spouse.

If the spouse is not the physician's patient, permission should be requested to call him or her. Such a request carries an obvious risk. It is best to avoid asking permission during the drinking history; the request should be made elsewhere in the interview. Also, the request should not be tied to the drinking issue but should be associated with an overall health concern. Finally, the physician should not risk destroying the relationship if excessive resistance is shown.

One approach which usually gets satisfactory results is to say casually, near the end of the interview, "By the way, I hope you won't mind if I call your wife (husband) to see if she (he) can help me learn a bit more about the problem." Of course, a refusal at this point may be fruitfully discussed at a later interview.

While a spouse or other family member is usually a reliable informant, the physician should be aware that he may receive a distorted account in a few instances. Occasionally the informant is an abstainer, has strong feelings against any alcohol use and considers the mere fact of consumption to be a drinking problem. Such a person will be unable to offer any substantial evidence of adverse behavioral consequences beyond his own upset at the sight of the individual drinking.

More commonly, an informant may appear to be covering up a patient's drinking problem. Such informants may do so because: (1) they are ashamed to be related to an alcoholic; (2) they mistakenly believe they are helping by denying that there is a problem; (3) they have a pathologic need to keep the person dependent, or (4) they also have an alcohol problem. When dealing with the first two reasons, the physician can usually penetrate the denial with some educational efforts. However, he will most often be frustrated, regardless of the strategy he uses, when facing the latter two reasons.

In rural areas, physicians sometimes have a distinct advantage in being able to utilize the best of all sources of information— common knowledge, or town gossip. Thus, the various strategies for eliciting information become superfluous, because the physician could complete the drinking history without talking to the individual. Unfortunately, in many cases this diagnostic advantage is offset by potential complications in the treatment phase. Certainly the interview strategies discussed in this article will be of greater value to those physicians practicing in the relative anonymity of urban settings.

Chapter 10

PSYCHOSEXUAL ADJUSTMENT AND COUNSELING AFTER MYOCARDIAL INFARCTION

MICHAEL MCLANE, HARRY KROP AND JAWAHAR MEHTA

The critical nature and widespread prevalence of coronary heart disease have made it the focus of considerable attention in recent years, particularly regarding rehabilitation of patients who have had myocardial infarctions. With mortality from myocardial infarction on the decline (1), the responsibility of providing the patient with the means to facilitate his or her rehabilitation becomes even greater. The goal of cardiac rehabilitation has come to be viewed by many as extending and improving the quality of life by restoring and maintaining the patient at his or her optimal level of physiologic, psychologic, emotional, vocational, social, and economic usefulness compatible with the patient's functional capacity. This approach has stimulated numerous studies on comprehensive programs associated with the rehabilitation of patients recovering from myocardial infarction.

PROBLEMS IN PSYCHOSEXUAL ADJUSTMENT

Survivors of myocardial infarction and their families are forced to make significant social and psychological adjustments. The course of cardiac recovery is marked by a number of psychological problems (2). Depression and anxiety are commonly exhibited for periods up to 1 year and are at times accompanied by irritability, exhaustion, boredom, and feelings of hopelessness. Because

Reprinted with permission from *Annals of Internal Medicine*, 92: 514-19, 1980.

patients are weak and easily fatigue when they first arrive home from the hospital, they often see themselves as potential invalids or in a state of "cardiac decline." Frequently, this depression is masked but is characterized by sense of loss, preoccupation with the future, fear of falling asleep, and a host of anxiety-related physical symptoms.

The individual patient is not the only victim of a heart attack; families suffer as well. Spouses, for example, report increased anxiety, depression, psychosomatic symptoms (including chest pain and palpitations), sleep and appetite disturbances, and marital tension (3). Typically, the spouse finds it difficult to strike a balance between being helpful and allowing the patient to return to an appropriate level of activity. Adsett and Bruhn (4) reported that the wives of their cardiac patients were generally overprotective of their husbands or were afraid to make demands on them, to upset them emotionally, or to allow them to participate in many physical activities. Additionally, they stated that many of the wives experienced guilt about their spouses' heart disease and frequently questioned themselves as to what they might have done to contribute to the cardiac episodes. The authors also remarked that the wives of patients suffered marked inhibition in their expression of hostility. Wives may become overly solicitous to their husbands after myocardial infarction (5). The entire family, including children, may treat the patient in this manner (6, 7). With both the patients and the family suffering from symptoms of depression and anxiety, serious conflicts in the family may occur during the first few months after an acute myocardial infarction regardless of the stability of the relationship before the event (8).

Krop and his associates (2) studied 100 married male patients at a Veterans Administration Hospital to determine what concerns the patients might have regarding their recovery and how well these concerns were being communicated. The subjects were given an extensive questionnaire on the day of discharge from the hospital that pertained to demographic, medical, social, and sexual history before hospitalization and to their fears or concerns about social, vocational, and sexual aspects of their future. Fifty-one percent expressed concerns that their marital relationship would be considerably affected by their cardiac condition. In contrast, only 11% reported being concerned before the myocardial infarction. In a study of 24 married patients (8), Wishnie and colleagues found that 18 were anxious or depressed enough to require medication, 15 had sleep disturbances, and 18 had serious marital conflicts during the first 3 months after myocardial infarction. The authors pointed out that most conflicts hinge on misunderstanding of the coronary disease and on misinterpreting the physician's orders. Skelton and Dominian (9) investigated the psychological consequences of myocardial infarction in 65 wives of husbands admitted to a cardiac care unit and found that 38% had a high degree of stress characterized by feelings of loss, guilt, and depression. Twenty-seven percent reported an appreciable change in their marital relationships as a result of increased tension, irritability, and anxiety of both partners. This tension was noted especially during the convalescent period. Additionally, the wives of coronary patients suffer the same fears, lack of knowledge, and misconceptions as their husbands do (10). Major changes in lifelong roles may be another stress on the marital relationship (3). The wife may be forced to become the major means of economic support for the family, often after many years as a homemaker. Likewise, the husband may find responsibilities as a homemaker an additional stress when the wife suffers a myocardial infarction.

The high incidence of marital conflict makes it crucial that it be considered an important aspect of the rehabilitation process. Yet, it is evident that this has been neglected by many physicians in the hospital. Krop and associates (2) pointed out that of their patients who had marital concerns, only 15% discussed them with their physicians, and most of these discussions were initiated by the patient himself. These findings support the observations of Amsterdam and co-workers (11), who studied resumption of sexual activity after myocardial infarction and concluded that despite patients' desires for counseling on marital and sexual matters, their needs were not being adequately met by physicians. In the Boston Veterans Administration study (12), a discrepancy between the patient and the physician's perception of the frequency of discussions about "intimate issues" was evident. Patients perceived doctors as initiating discussions of sex and marriage much less frequently than physicians thought they did, although both agreed that patients seldom initiated discussions of sex unless they have psychiatric illness. Conceivably, physicians themselves are not clear as to how to handle such discussions.

QUANTITY AND QUALITY OF SEXUAL FUNCTIONING AFTER MYOCARDIAL INFARCTION

A major area of frequent concern within marital relationships is sexuality. Sex is generally not widely discussed between the husband and wife. This may be related to myths that center around sex and the cardiac patient. This communication gap is further exacerbated by the physician's own discomfort about discussing sex. Consequently, the patient leaves the hospital with concerns that have not been addressed or for which the patient has received only vague information. Thus, often the couple is left with the responsibility of deciding what is correct. The detrimental effects of coronary heart disease on sexual functioning can be seen most readily by the decline in the quality and quantity of sexual activity. The decrease in quantity or frequency has been repeatedly demonstrated. One study (12) showed a 58% decrease in sexual activity in patients who had suffered a coronary event. In the 6-month follow-up period, a decline in frequency of orgasms from 2.1 to 1.6 per week was noted. Similar findings were described by Bloch and colleagues (13) in a study of 100 patients after myocardial infarction. A decrease of 48% in sexual intercourse based on a premorbid monthly mean of 5.2 to a mean of 2.7 11 months later was reported.

In a retrospective study (11), 43% of patients had decreased frequency of or abstinence from sexual intercourse. Johnston and associates (14) found a significant decrease in absolute frequency of sexual intercourse from 6.5 to 4.6 times per month before and after the cardiac event. The mean follow-up period was 47 months after myocardial infarction. In another study in similar patients (9), 26 of 38 couples were having sexual intercourse less frequently 3 months after myocardial infarction, but most of these couples began to return to their pre-illness pattern about 1 year later. Klein and co-workers (15) reported that 15 out of 20 patients with a history of myocardial infarction claimed either abstinence or diminished sexual activity.

In addition to a decrease in frequency, a serious decline in the quality of sexual activity is often seen in patients with myocardial infarction, (8, 16). The commonest problems reported by male patients are decreased sexual desire and impotence. Tuttle and colleagues (16) interviewed male patients in a work-evaluation clinic and found that in addition to a general reduction in the frequency of sexual activity, 10% reported permanent impotence. In a study designed to investigate the long-term effects of myocardial infarction on marital and sexual functioning (17), we found that 37% of patients had premature ejaculation, 54% manifested retarded ejaculation, and 60% had erectile difficulties at least half of the time. Abromov (18), in one of the few studies to evaluate the sexual activity of female patients, found sexual frigidity and dissatisfaction in 65% of subjects as compared to 24% of age-matched controls who were hospitalized for reasons other than cardiac problems.

In reviewing the studies conducted on the postmyocardial infarction patient, we have ascertained three major areas that need to be considered in determining sexual activity: physiologic factors, psycholsocial adjustment, and drug effects.

Physiological Factors

Most experts agree that there are few, if any physiologic reasons for the cardiac patient not to achieve sexual satisfaction (19). Douglas and Wilkes (20) gave support to this idea by using a measure of oxygen consumption. They found that the average energy cost for foreplay was 3.5 metabolic equivalents (mets) and for orgasm, in the range of 4.7 to 5.5 mets. Since most patients with uncomplicated myocardial infarction are capable of 8 to 9 mets (21), Douglas and Wilkes concluded that sexual activity is well within the capacity of most cardiac patients. Hellerstein and Friedman (22) have shown that the average expenditure of energy in sexual intercourse is about 3.7 mets, while the average expenditure for most everyday tasks is 5 to 6 mets. These investigators also compared the average heart rate achieved at orgasm to that for most occupational activities, and found that the maximal rate achieved during orgasm (mean, 117 beats/min) was similar to that achieved during other occupational activities (120 beats/min). Nemec and co-authors (23) have also reported an average heart rate during orgasm of 114 ±14 beats/min for the male superior position and 117 ± 14 beats/min for the female superior position. Bruce and co-workers (24) studied heart rates in 495 patients with stable angina and after myocardial infarction and found that the maximum heart rate achieved in their patients before development of symptoms was 145 ± 23 beats/min, which on comparison to a heart rate of 117 beats/min at orgasm represents only 81% of their predicted maximum capacity. Determination of exercise capability soon after myocardial infarction may help provide information as to whether a given patient can attain a heart rate of 115 to 120 beats/min without symptoms. If the rate achieved is lower, a further convalescent period and a retesting of exercise capability may provide a scientific basis for encouraging sexual rehabilitation.

The patient's physiologic limitations due to coronary heart disease must be clearly known before a plan for resuming sexual activity can be formulated. This plan must be individualized, and limiting factors such as chest pain, dyspnea, or palpitations must be considered. Because of individual limiting factors, it is difficult to say how long after myocardial infarction a patient should wait before returning to sexual function. Some suggest a waiting period of about 6 weeks, whereas others (25) advise the resumption of sexual activity when the patient is able to climb one or two flights of stairs or walk several blocks at a brisk pace. Masturbation could also be a gradual means of returning to sexual activity. It may also be possible to improve the patient's limitations through physical conditioning programs.

Psychosocial Adjustment

Another important factor leading to sexual dysfunction after myocardial infarction is the psychological condition of the patient. Cardiac patients and their spouses frequently suffer feelings of depression, anxiety, and fears about a relapse or sudden death. These feelings, along with cardiac symptoms (that is, chest pain and fatigability) and the spouse's reluctance to engage in sex, are reasons most often given for the decreased sexual activity (13). Recent studies have been shown that depression and anxiety may affect sexual libido profoundly. Stern and associates (26) studied 63 patients who had suffered myocardial infarction. They found that 13% were still depressed or anxious 1 year after the event and that these patients had markedly lower rates of sexual functioning. In a study of the psychological consequences suffered by the wives of such patients, Skelton and Dominian (9) observed that of 65 patients with a history of myocardial infarction, 28 suffered anxiety and depression, and 26 either had not resumed intercourse after 3 months or were doing so less frequently. Hellerstein and Friedman (27) also reported that of 48 similar patients, 17 had a change in sexual desire, a fear of intercourse, or were depressed. When depression or anxiety is prominent in either or both the patient and the spouse, it can affect sexual activity. The wife may find that she is unable to enjoy sex because of anxieties about her husband's condition, and this may, in turn, produce feelings of sexual inadequacy in the patient, thereby further exacerbating his psychological condition.

Much of the psychological difficulty experienced by the recovering cardiac patient may be related to the absence of adequate information on resumption of normal activities (2, 17, 28). This is particularly true in the case of sexual functioning, which has traditionally not been addressed by health-care professionals despite the general acceptance that providing specific information to the patient is desirable (29). Perhaps sexual counseling and explaining that sex usually does not impose excessive demands on the heart may prevent psychogenic sexual problems in the future. Part of this communication deficit may exist because the patient and spouse are usually uncomfortable about relating these personal, nonmedical problems to the busy physician. These sensitive and emotional problems tend to be discussed only when they are uncovered by the health-care professional through specific questioning (8). The largest share of the responsibility for this communication gap must be borne by the physician, who is often embarrassed by the subject, conservative in giving advice, or unknowledgeable about the subject (30). There is indeed a lack of information available to clinicians on sexual functioning of cardiac patients (31, 32). Elimination of this problem can only be done through informed discussion of the return to sexual functioning by the patient, spouse, physician, and an expert in sexual counseling.

An important psychological consideration is the manner in

which the recovering patient copes with his condition. Most noticeable are two maladaptive coping styles, the "denier" and the "cardiac invalid." The former has a strong tendency to overdo everything in an effort to prove he is not handicapped by his condition. He will often refuse to comply with medical advice about his diet, medication, physical activity, and return to work. This patient will typically refuse to give up undesirable habits such as smoking and drinking and will discount his fear of death. The latter type of recovering cardiac patient may experience features of invalidism, the opposite of the denial coping style. The patient may come to harbor the constant care and attention given to him in the early stages of recovery. This excessive helplessness may develop into the patient's primary means of social interaction and gratification. This coping style may also hold economic stability in cases where the patient receives a disability income related to his cardiac condition. The result is deconditioning and physical inactivity that commonly lead to weakness, shortness of breath, and tachycardia (33), which further convince the patient that he really is an invalid. Both maladaptive coping styles are the result of not being able to respond to crisis by working through the normal processes, which often are accompanied by unacceptable feelings of anger, disbelief, helplessness, depression, fear, and denial. Naturally, the sexual functioning of the patient is affected by these coping patterns. The "denier" often tries to reaffirm his masculinity through hypersexuality, which, in turn, may increase the spouse's anxiety about her husband's capacity. Consistent with his belief about his disabled status, the "cardiac invalid" will exhibit the opposite behavior and drastically reduce or abstain from sexual intercourse altogether. Both of these extremes serve to further impede and complicate the rehabilitation process. Indications are that some patients who have serious marital or sexual difficulties before myocardial infarction will use their invalid status to avoid sexual intimacy. This underscores the need to accurately assess premorbid sexual functioning before developing a rehabilitation program.

There are two myths about sexuality important to the study of the recovering cardiac patient. First is the popular belief that a person suffering from an illness should not be sexually active.

This myth probably evolves from the general feeling that one must become physically inactive and psychologically passive during recovery from illness. This aspect of the "sick role" denies the patient the fulfillment of a basic need that may even be therapeutic in its effect. Myths about sudden death during sexual intercourse are widespread, and in fact the patient's belief in these can contribute dramatically to the decline in sexual activity (16, 17, 22). To a patient not properly informed, it may seem logical that sexual activity would tax the heart beyond its capacity. Further, there are only a few cardiac rehabilitation programs that include information on resumption of sexual activities. Actual reported cases of myocardial infarction during coitus are rare and are usually associated with additional stress factors such as sex in the context of an extramarital affair or after heavy consumption of food or alcohol (34, 35). Ueno (36) investigated 5559 sudden deaths and found that only 18 (0.03%) were related to coitus, and that 14 of these were during extramarital intercourse. This might indicate that coital death is perhaps more related to stress than to sexual intercourse per se (19). Further evidence is presented by Scheingold and Wagner (37), who have reported that deaths during treadmill stress tests are generally much higher than those achieved during sexual intercourse. This evidence points to the need for specific counseling about the limitations of the cardiac patient and for correcting the misinformation he may hold.

Drugs as a Cause of Psychological and Sexual Dysfunction

Patients with myocardial infarction frequently are treated with medications that my result in sexual dysfunction. In additon, other often associated disease states such as diabetes mellitus and hypertension may result in sexual and psychological problems that the patient may relate to heart disease. Although a host of pharmacologic agents have been implicated in psychosexual dysfunctions, some of the more commonly used drugs need close attention. Very few patients will, of course, volunteer infor- mation about sexual difficulties. A good patient-physician rapport may bring out the association of drug therapy with the psychosexual problems in the individual.

Since normal sexual physiology requires adequate function of the autonomic nervous system, sexual dysfunction is common in the diabetic or hypertensive patient. Centrally mediated sympathetic outflow regulates potency, that is, achievement and maintenance of erection, whereas ejaculation and orgasm depend on peripheral sympathetic function. Centrally acting antihypertensive agents such as methyldopa, clonidine, and reserpine may affect potency in one third of recipients (38). Peripherally acting sympatholytic agents such as guanethidine may result in abnormalities of ejaculation in about two thirds of recipients. Secondarily, impotency may result as a psychological outcome. Drugs such as diuretics can also cause both impotence and failure of ejaculation in about one third of subjects (38, 39). The degree of sexual impairment may vary from patient to patient and is often dose dependent.

The beta blocker propranolol is commonly used in patients with previous myocardial infarction for a host of indications. Propranolol can impair sexual function, perhaps on a central basis. Although the prevalence of such side effects is believed to be low, a detailed sexual history may reveal the true prevalence. In a recent study designed to investigate sexual dysfunction in patients maintained on propranolol therapy (40), 15% developed impotence, 28% had decreased potency, and 4% had decreased libido. The severity of sexual dysfunction was related to the dose of propranolol used.

An evaluation of a patient's problems, manipulation of type and dose of offending agent, and trial with different drugs or combinations may be rewarding. When drug-induced impotence is intractable, sensitivity counseling, reassurance, and sexual therapy may be beneficial.

SEXUAL COUNSELING

Often patients who suffer myocardial infarction find they must come to terms with their vulnerability to illness and, perhaps for the first time, the realization of their mortality. The shock of this event may have effects that go much deeper than the medical problem itself. Most couples are not prepared to make the psychosocial adjustments necessary for functional recovery. If sexuality occupied an important place in the lives of these couples, then specific information on the return to sexual functioning should be included in the rehabilitation process.

It is important that physicians provide a sensitive and understanding atmosphere so that patients with sexual concerns will be sufficiently comfortable to express them. Some patients may use this opportunity to participate in sex counseling for longstanding difficulties in sexual intimacy or to convince the spouse to participate in this counseling. The physician must also recognize that some patients will not be able to introduce the topic of sex regardless of the quality of patient-physician communication and should be prepared to approach the subject as a matter of routine. Physicians should be aware that not all patients will have problems after myocardial infarction and some who report no sexual problems may be denying their existence. Any specific information must take into account the patient's sexual attitudes, premorbid sexual activity, age, and psychological condition in addition to his or her general health, frequency of pain or arrhythmias, and functional capacity. In addition, it is necessary to assess accurately the couple's premorbid sexual adaptation by addressing such variables as frequency of coitus, level of sexual desire, capacity for arousal, orgasmic experience, and sexual attitudes. A thorough sexual history can be invaluable in designing a program of behavioral changes within the relationship and will increase the likelihood that these changes will be beneficial and enduring for both partners.

The current trend in cardiac rehabilitation is toward a multidisciplinary approach, although the composition of the team may vary widely. Rehabilitation program formats also differ in modalities being used. An eclectic program of individual counseling has been used by the University of Texas Medical Branch to provide information and support to cardiac patients and their partners (41). A similar program of providing verbal information and support is advocated by Semmler and Semmler (42). Moore and associates (43) favor use of printed material developed from the questions of 30 cardiac patients. Group therapy is used in the outpatient management of cardiac patients at the Naval Hospital in San Diego (5). An audiovisual approach has been developed by the authors for patients at the Veterans Administration Medical Center in Gainesville, Florida. As with most new and independently developing programs, there remains a need to evaluate the comparative differences and similarities with regard to their effectiveness. It should be emphasized that there is no fixed style to the counseling of patients and their partners, but here are a number of basic similarities among rehabilitation programs. Most programs point out the importance of initiating the rehabilitation process as soon as the cardiac patient is medically stable. Whenever possible, the spouse's needs should be considered and therefore be included in the rehabilitation process. The information provided to the couple should be specific, accurate, and take into consideration the patient's physical status. The counselor should consider the couple's value system and similarly be aware of the patient's pre-illness, sexual attitudes, and activity. Perhaps most important, sexual counseling should be supportive and reassuring to the couple and should strive to facilitate communication between the patient and partner.

Although there is as yet no objective evidence of effectiveness of psychosocial counseling on the well-being of the patient and his or her family, it would seem that such intervention might be beneficial. We may have to wait some more years until data from several other studies have been accumulated before a definite answer is available.

APPENDIX

Case Histories

PATIENT 1: A 61-year-old married, retired veteran was hospitalized with his first myocardial infarction. On the ninth day of hospitalization, the patient completed a questionnaire that addressed possible sexual and marital concerns, and then he requested a private conference with one of the authors. He admitted that his foremost concern after learning he was not going to die was the future of his sexual relationship with his wife. He pointed out that since none of the doctors initiated the topic, he assumed that it was a "taboo" subject. He thought that he would never engage in sexual activities again. After discussion with his physician about the nature and severity of myocardial infarction, and a submaximal stress test, sexual counseling was initiated with him and his wife of 34 years, who also had (unexpressed) fears about her role as a sexual partner. After a sexual history was obtained from them, the physician provided information on the effects of cardiac disease on sexual functioning and of sexual functioning on cardiac disease. The couple was encouraged to share openly their fears and concerns with each other and was assured that some degree of stress associated with the rehabilitation process is normal. It was impressed upon them that readjustment requires understanding and some degree of experimentation by both partners. The patient and his wife were also given a set of specific sexual exercises (for example, sensate focus) to assure a gradual re-establishment of comfortable sexual patterns. At 6-month follow-up, the patient and his wife showed an excellent adjustment and a return to healthy sexual functioning.

PATIENT 2: A 52-year-old lawyer was hospitalized after his first myocardial infarction. From our interviews with him, it was clear that his sexual relationship with his wife of 3 years was very unsatisfactory. Although eager to discuss his dissatisfaction, the patient was reluctant to consider counseling because "my wife wouldn't be interested." He added that "having a heart attack clinches my going the rest of my life without sex." After further discussions with him, it was clear that he had been impotent for the past 7 years and had ceased all attempts to initiate sexual activity 4 years before his heart attack. It also became apparent that he perceived his inability to financially support his wife as proof of "my being only half a man."

Before discharge from the hospital, he reluctantly gave us permission to bring up the sexual issue during the exit interview with him and his wife. He was surprised and pleased when his wife responded with total support. Both agreed to enter sex therapy after discharge. The authors counseled this couple for seven sessions successfully using a Masters and Johnson approach. A 6-month follow-up not only indicated that the couple had satisfactorily adjusted after myocardial infarction, but also that they had developed a more satisfying marital and sexual relationship than they had experienced at any time during their marriage. This case illustrates the precipitation of sexual problems by myocardial infarction and shows that intervention soon thereafter may be beneficial.

REFERENCES

1. *Heart Facts*, Dallas: American Heart Association, 1979.

2. H. Krop, D. Hall, and J. Mehta, Sexual concerns after myocardial infarction. *Sex Disability, 2:*91-7, 1971.
3. C. M. Cole, E. M. Levin, and N. Holcomb, Psychosocial aspects of cardiac rehabilitation. *Proceedings of the Conference on Cardiac Rehabilition Following Infarction.* Galveston, TX: University of Texas Press, 1978, p. 8.
4. C. A. Adsett and J. G. Bruhn, Short-term group psychotherapy for post-myocardial infarction patients and their wives. *Can Med Assoc J, 99:* 577-84, 1968.
5. R. H. Rahe et al., Group therapy in the outpatient management of post-myocardial infarction patients. *Psychiatry Med, 4:*77-88, 1973.
6. R. White and S. Liddon, Ten survivors of cardiac arrest. *Psychiatry Med, 3:*219-25, 1972.
7. A. Cobb, *Medical and Psychological Aspects of Disability.* Springfield: Thomas, 1973, pp. 8-70.
8. H. A. Wishnie, T. P. Hackett, and N. H. Cassem, Psychological hazards of convalescence following myocardial infarction. *JAMA, 215:*1292-6, 1971.
9. M. Skelton and J. Dominian, Psychological stress in wives of patients with myocardial infarction. *British Med J, 2:*101-3, 1973.
10. J. E. Crawshaw, Community rehabilitation after acute myocardial infarction. *Heart Lung, 3:*258-62, 1974.
11. E. A. Amsterdam et al., Sexual counseling and sexual activity after myocardial infarction: patient attitudes and physician response. *Clin Res, 25:* 86A, 1977.
12. C. A. Pinderhughes et al., Interrelationships between sexual functioning and medical conditions. *Med Aspects Hum Sex, 6:*52-75, 1975.
13. A. Bloch, J. Maeder, and J. Haisley, Sexual problems after myocardial infarction. *Am Heart J, 90:*536-7, 1972.
14. B. L. Johnston et al., Sexual activity in exercising patients after myocardial infarction and revascularization. *Heart Lung, 7:*1026-31, 1978.
15. R. F. Klein et al., The physician and postmyocardial invalidism. *JAMA, 194:* 143-8, 1965.
16. W. B. Tuttle, W. L. Cook, and E. Fitche, Sexual behavior in post-myocardial infarction patients. *Am J Cardiol, 13:*140, 1964.
17. J. Mehta and H. D. Krop, The effect of myocardial infarction on sexual functioning. *Sex Disability, 2:*115-20, 1979.
18. L. A. Abramov, Sexual life and sexual frigidity among women developing acute myocardial infarction. *Psychosom Med, 38:*418-25, 1976.
19. C. Bakker, M. Bogdonoff, and H. Hellerstein, Heart disease and sex response to questions. *Med Aspects Hum Sex, 5:*24-35, 1971.
20. J. E. Douglas and T. D. Wilkes, Reconditioning cardiac patients. *Am Fam Physician, 11:*123-9, 1975.
21. R. S. Elliot and R. Miles, Brief guide to office counseling; advising the cardiac patient about sexual intercourse. *Med Aspects Hum Sex, 9:* 49-50, 1975.

22. H. K. Hellerstein and E. H. Friedman, Sexual activity and the post-coronary patient. *Med Aspects Hum Sex, 3:*70-96, 1969.
23. E. D. Nemec, L. Mansfield, and J. W. Kennedy, Heart rate and blood pressure responses during sexual activity in normal males. *Am Heart J, 92:*274-7, 1976.
24. R. A. Bruce et al., Separation of effects of cardiovascular disease and age on ventricular function with maximal exercise. *Am J Cardiol, 34:* 757-63, 1974.
25. M. A. Abbott and D. P. McWhirter, Resuming sexual activity after myocardial infarction. *Med Aspects Hum Sex, 12:*18-29, 1978.
26. M. J. Stern, L. Pascale, and J. B. McLoone, Psychosocial adaptation following an acute myocardial infarction. *J Clin Dis, 29:*513-26, 1974.
27. H. K. Hellerstein and E. H. Friedman, Sexual activity and the post-coronary patient. *Arch Intern Med, 125:*987-99, 1970.
28. R. Nagle, R. Gangola, and I. Picton-Robinson, Factors influencing return to work after myocardial infarction. *Lancet, 2:*454-6, 1971.
29. W. D. Gentry and R. B. Williams, *Psychological Aspects of Myocardial Infarction and Coronary Care.* St. Louis: C. V. Mosby, 1975, pp. 112-7.
30. J. M. Friedman, Sexual adjustment of the post-coronary male. In J. LoPiccolo and M. LoPiccolo (Eds.), *Handbook of Sex Therapy.* New York: Plenum, 1978, p. 375.
31. A. M. McGill, *Review of Literature on Cardiovascular Rehabilitation: Proceedings of the National Heart and Lung Institute Working Conference on Behavior.* Washington D. C.: U. S. Government Printing Office, 1975.
32. L. Jacobson, Illness and human sexuality. *Neuro Outlook, 22:*50-3, 1974.
33. N. Wenger, *Coronary Care: Rehabilitation After Myocardial Infarction.* New York: American Heart Association, 1973, p. 5.
34. G. X. Trimble, The coital coronary. *Med Aspects Hum Sex, 4:*64-72, 1970.
35. E. Massie, E. Rose, and R. Whelton, Sudden death during coitus: fact or fiction? *Med Aspects Hum Sex, 3:*22-6, 1969.
36. M. Ueno, The so-called coital death. *Japanese J Leg Med, 17:*535, 1963.
37. L. P. Scheingold and N. N. Wagner, *Sound Sex and the Aging Heart.* New York: Human Sciences Press, 1974, p. 89.
38. M. J. Reichgott, Problems of sexual function in patients with hypertension. *Cardiovasc Med, 4:*149-56, 1979.
39. J. G. Douglas, J. W. Hollifield, and G. W. Liddle, Treatment of longrenin essential hypertension: comparison of spironolactone and a hydro-chlorothiazide-triamterne combination. *JAMA, 227:*518-21, 1974.
40. W. C. Burnett and R. A. Chahine, Sexual dysfunction as a complication of propranolol therapy in men. *Cardiovasc Med, 4:*811-5, 1979.
41. C. M. Cole, A treatment strategy for postmyocardial sexual dysfunction. *Sex Disability, 2:*122-9, 1979.
42. C. Semmler and M. Semmler, Counseling the coronary patient. *Am J Occup Ther, 28:*609-13, 1974.
43. K. Moore, M. Folk-Lighty, and M. J. Nolen, The joy of sex after a heart attack: counseling the cardiac patient. *Nursing, 7:*53-5, 1977.

Chapter 11

DOCTOR-PATIENT COMMUNICATION IN PATIENTS WITH ARTHRITIS

D. M. GRENNAN, SUSAN TAYLOR AND D. G. PALMER

INTRODUCTION

The difficulties involved in patient-doctor communication have been emphasised in a number of previous studies (Butt, 1977: Joyce and others, 1969; Kirscht, 1977). Drug therapy, although helpful in terms of relief from pain and stiffness, is not curative in patients with rheumatic diseases (Brooks, Buchanan, 1976) and although all would not accept the viewpoint that communication may be the only form of treatment there is (Joyce and others, 1969), it is obviously of particular importance. Patients with chronic arthritides may take simple analgesic drugs, non-steroidal anti-inflammatory (NSAI) drugs such as salicylates or indomethacin, or more potentially effective drugs such as gold salts or penicillamine for a number of years. The results expected from therapy with these two groups of drugs differ in that first-line anti-inflammatory compounds can only be expected to produce symptomatic relief of pain and stiffness while gold and penicillamine are given on a long-term basis in an effort to supress the underlying disease process. The potential side effects of these two groups of drugs also differ, the former group commonly producing gastrointestinal irritation and possibly ulceration while the latter group has the potential of producing more serious toxic side effects such as bone marrow suppression and renal toxicity, which may be heralded by less serious side effects such as sore mouths, pruritus or rashes. It

Reprinted with permission from *The New Zealand Medical Journal*, 87:431-4, 1978.

would thus seem particularly desirable that patients being treated with these drugs should have some knowledge of the symptoms of their potential side effects and also of the realistic aims of therapy.

In this survey, a group of 50 patients who had a well-defined, chronic form of arthritis were presented with a standard questionnaire concerned with their knowledge of their disease, the drugs they were taking and the aims of therapy. A non-medical interviewer who had not played a part in their management (S.T.) undertook the interview.

METHODS

PATIENTS. Forty-six consecutive outpatients with a well-defined arthritic condition (rheumatoid arthritis, ankylosing spondylitis or osteoarthritis) who were receiving drugs for their arthritis and four patients who had been admitted to the rheumatic diseases ward during the study period were interviewed. The patients with rheumatoid arthritis (36) all satisfied the criteria of the American Rheumatism Association for a diagnosis of definite or classical rheumatoid arthritis (Ropes and others, 1958) and the patients with ankylosing spondylitis (5) satisfied diagnostic criteria of the W. H. O. (1963). The patients with osteoarthritis (9) all had at least Grade 3 radiological changes of osteoarthritis (W. H. O., 1963a) together with symptoms attributable to their osteoarthritis.

The ages of the patients ranged from 20 years to 81 years (mean 52 years). Fourteen were male. The duration of disease varied from six months to 36 years (mean 11.6 years).

INTERVIEW. A standard questionnaire was used. The interview was carried out by S. T. in a private room and in the absence of medical personnel. Questions relating to each topic were put to each patient in simple non-medical language and in a standard fashion for every patient. Details of the questionnaire may be obtained from the author.

RESULTS

The details of the patients in the different disease categories are shown in Table XI-1. All but four of the patients were cooperative and happy to take part in the survey. However, four patients

TABLE XI-1
DETAILS OF DIFFERENT PATIENT CATEGORIES

	Rheumatoid Arthritis	Ankylosing Spondylitis	Osteoarthritis
Number of patients	36	5	9
Number of males	8	5	1
Number of females	28	0	8
Age range (years)	20 to 74	25 to 48	57 to 81
Mean age (years)	56	35	66
Range of duration of disease (years)	0.5 to 34	5 to 20	3 to 25
Mean duration of disease (years)	11.5	9.2	14.0
Range of age of onset of disease (years)	17 to 60	17 to 33	26 to 78
Mean age of onset of disease (years)	44	26	52

appeared resentful either of their disease or its failure to respond to therapy. Three of these patients had a severe deforming rheumatoid arthritis and one mild and early ankylosing spondylitis but in addition a previous history of personality disorder.

KNOWLEDGE OF DISEASE. Forty-three of the 50 patients knew the type of arthritis from which they suffered. Thirty-two of 37 patients (87 percent) who were more than 52 years of age and 11 of 13 patients (85 percent) who were less than 53 years knew the diagnosis. In the different patient categories 86 percent of patients with rheumatoid arthritis, 80 percent with ankylosing spondylitis and 89 percent with osteoarthritis were aware of the correct diagnosis although only six patients with rheumatoid arthritis (16 percent) volunteered the fact that this was an inflammatory disease with tendency towards remission and exacerbation.

DRUG NAME RECALL. Thirty-seven of the 50 patients overall knew the names of the particular anti-arthritic drugs which they were taking. In the particular patient categories 25 of the 36 patients with rheumatoid, all of the nine patients with osteo-arthritis and three of the five patients with ankylosing spondylitis knew the drugs they were taking.

Twenty-seven of the 35 patients (75 percent) over 52 years and 10 of the 14 patients (71 percent) under 53 years knew the names of the different drugs they were taking. Eighteen of the 20 patients (90 percent) with a disease duration of longer than 12 years and 19 of the 30 patients (63 percent) with a disease duration of longer than 12 years knew this information. These differences were not statistically significant.

AWARENESS OF DRUG SIDE EFFECTS. All but two patients overall were receiving non-steroidal anti-inflammatory or simple analgesic drugs while of the rheumatoid patients, five were also receiving penicillamine, gold or an immunosuppressive drug and eight were receiving oral corticosteroids.

Thirty-two of 44 (73 percent) patients receiving NSAI drugs did not mention gastro-intestinal symptoms when asked about possible side effects of these drugs. Five of these 32 patients who were receiving either salicylate preparations or indomethacin mentioned dizziness or ringing in the ears as possible side effects, two who were receiving salicylates mentioned the possibility of renal side effects and one who was receiving phenylbutazone mentioned the possibility of an effect on the white blood cells. Fifteen of the 32 patients were receiving either soluble aspirin or indomethacin only. Overall, of the patients receiving NSAI drugs six of the 13 patients aged under 53 years (46 percent) and six of 31 patients (19 percent) aged over 52 years knew that gastro-intestinal symptoms were possible side effects of their drugs. These differences were not statistically significant at the 0.05 level when analysed by the Chi-squared test.

On the other hand only four of the 13 patients with rheumatoid arthritis who were receiving the potentially more toxic "second-line" group of anti-rheumatic drugs (penicillamine, gold or immunosuppressive drugs) had some idea of the symptoms which might signify drug toxicity. All these four patients were aged less than 56 years (there were five rheumatoid patients under 56 years who were receiving these drugs overall). None of the eight rheumatoid patients older than 56 years of age who were receiving these drugs had any idea of their potential side effects or of their toxicity. These differences were statistically significant when analysed by Fischer's Exact Test (P>0.01).

THERAPEUTIC EXPECTATIONS. Patients were also asked if they thought their drugs would cure their arthritis. Of the 32 patients with rheumatoid arthritis receiving the non-steroidal anti-inflammatory drugs only three thought this was likely to be the case. None of the seven patients with osteoarthritis and only one of the five patients with ankylosing spondylitis who were receiving non-steroidal anti-inflammatory drugs or simple analgesics thought these could cure their disease. Only one of the 12 patients with rheumatoid arthritis receiving "second-line" anti-rheumatic drugs thought these drugs would cure their arthritis.

Forty patients overall said that they were taking all the drugs which were prescribed for them. Six of the ten patients who were not taking the drugs they had been advised to take confessed they had not admitted this to their physician. Thus in at least five out of 36 patients (14 percent) with rheumatoid arthritis and one of the five patients (20 percent) with ankylosing spondylitis the doctor thought they were receiving "second-line" anti-inflammatory drugs all affirmed that they were taking these drugs as directed.

Forty-four of the 50 patients (88 percent) thought that their drugs were helping them. Twenty-two of the 34 patients (65 percent) with rheumatoid arthritis, three of the nine patients (33 percent) with osteoarthritis and three of the five patients (60 percent) with ankylosing spondylitis thought their drugs had enabled them to stay at work or to continue to look after their families. Two of the six patients who thought that their drugs were not helping them were actually receiving "second-line" anti-inflammatory drugs.

DISCUSSION

Although only about 10 percent of sufferers from either inflammatory of degenerative arthritis will become totally disabled by their disease, most will have continued symptoms over a number of years (Duthie, 1957). The degree of disability which will develop is dependent not only upon disease severity but also upon adaptation to disease chronicity and a realistic awareness of the therapeutic expectations of anti-rheumatic drugs. The role of the physician with many of these patients has been said to "help the patients to help themselves" and to act as a "friend and counsellor" of the individual patient over a variable time period. In this situation in which patients are affected by a disease over many years it would seem particularly desirable that these patients should have some idea of the nature of their disease and in the inflammatory arthritis, its tendency to follow an intermittent course with remissions and exacerbations. It would also seem desirable that patients who may be taking either NSAI drugs over a number of years with a significant risk of producing gastric ulceration or drugs such as gold or penicillamine which pose even more serious side effects should have some idea of the side effects of these drugs might produce. In this study patients with an established form of either an inflammatory arthritis (rheumatoid arthritis or ankylosing spondylitis) or osteoarthritis were questioned in order to assess their understanding of their disease and of the drugs they had been prescribed. The interviewer was careful to ask the questions in a standardized "neutral" fashion designed not to lead the answer. Although over 80 percent of the patients interviewed knew from what form of joint disease they suffered only about 16 percent of patients with rheumatoid arthritis were aware that their disease was one of joint inflammation with a tendency towards natural remission and exacerbation. Thirteen of the patients did not know the names of the anti-rheumatic drugs which they were taking despite the fact that specific labelling of medicines in New Zealand has been a legal requirement for more than 10 years. There were no significant differences between the different disease catagories and different age groups in regard to this particular knowledge.

Furthermore, of the 44 patients receiving simple anti-inflammatory drugs only about one-quarter seemed aware that these drugs had potential gastro-intestinal side effects. This fact was especially relevant in that about half the patients who were unaware of this particular side effect were receiving either soluble aspirin or indomethacin which are amongst the more important drugs causing this side effect (Brooks, Buchanan, 1976). One might argue that the others who were receiving enteric-coated or delayed-release forms of salicylates or different types of proprionic acid derivative, were less likely to have gastro-intestinal side effects but it should be remembered that all of the simple anti-inflammatory drugs including ibuprofen, which is probably the safest in this respect, are able to cause peptic ulceration in susceptible patients. Because of the additional possibility of haematological toxicity the restricted use of phenylbutazone (only one patient) in this survey was reassuring. Nevertheless although aware of its potential haematological side effects, this patient was unaware of the ulcerogenic risk that is associated with this drug (Mason, Hayter, 1958). Fewer of the older patients than of the younger age group were aware of the possible side effects from anti-inflammatory drugs although these differences were not statistically significant.

Of greater importance, however, was the fact that none of the older patients with rheumatoid arthritis who were receiving the potentially more hazardous group of second-line anti-rheumatic drugs (gold or penicillamine) were able to volunteer any of the symptoms which would warn of their possible side effects while all but one of the five younger rheumatoid patients receiving this type of therapy were able to do so. This lack of knowledge in the older patients occurred despite repeated previous verbal instructions about possible side effects. The potential toxicity of gold is well known but was particularly emphasised by the findings of Girdwood (1974) that per million prescriptions, gold was the greatest single reported cause of drug deaths over a three-year period in the United Kingdom. Our own and others' experience with penicillamine (Multicentre Trial Group, 1971) suggests that this is little less toxic. Minor symptoms such as pruritus, a sore throat or sore mouth, may herald drug toxicity in patients receiving these drugs and it is important that such patients should know to report such symptoms to their doctor as soon as they are noticed. The importance of age in the retention of information has been noted in a previous study of patient-doctor communication in patients with arthritis (Joyce and others, 1969). Written aids to memory have been found to improve drug compliance in the elderly in other studies (Wandless, Davie, 1977) and such written aids would seem essential with respect to reporting of side effects in any elderly patients receiving potentially toxic remedies such as those discussed here.

REFERENCES

1. P. M. Brooks and W. W. Buchanan., Current management of rheumatoid arthritis. In W. W. Buchanan and W. C. Dick (Eds.), *Recent Advances in Rheumatology*. Edinburgh: Churchill Livingstone, 1976, Part Two, 32-87.

2. H. R. Butt, A method for better physician-patient communication. *Ann Intern Med. 86:*478-80, 1977.

3. J. J. R. Duthie, *Testbook of Rheumatic Diseases.* Edinburgh: Churchill Livingston, 1957, p. 259.
4. R. H. Girdwood, Death after taking medicaments. *British Med J, 1:*501-504, 1974.
5. C. R. B. Joyce, et al. Quantitative study of doctor-patient communication. *Q J Med, 38:*183-94, 1969.
6. J. P. Kirscht, Communication between patients and physicians. *Ann Intern Med, 86:*499-500, 1977.
7. R. M. Mason and R. R. P. Hayter, The present status of phenelbutazone therapy in rheumatic disease. *Practitioner, 181:*23-28, 1958.
8. Multicentre Trial Group, Controlled trial of D-penicillamine in severe rheumatoid arthritis. *Lancet, 1:*275-80, 1973.
9. M. W. Ropes et al., 1958 revision of diagnostic criteria for rheumatoid arthritis. *Bull Rheum Dis, 9:*175-6, 1958.
10. I. Wandless and J. W. Davie, Can drug compliance in the elderly be improved? *British Med J, 1:*359-61, 1977.
11. WHO, Proposed diagnostic criteria for use in population studies. In J. H. Kellgren, M. R. Jeffry, and J. Ball (Eds.), *The Epidemiology of Chronic Rheumatism,* Vol. 1. Oxford: Blackwell Scientific Publications, 1963, p. 326.
12. WHO, Atlas of standard radiographs of arthritis. In Kellgren, Jeffry, and Ball, *op. cit.,* vol. 2, p. 1.

Chapter 12

IMPORTANCE OF COMMUNICATION IN COUNSELLING THE SPINAL CORD INJURY PATIENT

VICTOR M. SANTANA CARLOS

INTRODUCTION

The considerable development in human services, particularly as regards interpersonal relations in the various types of communication, may be considered a manifest sign of a deep and rapid evolution—or should we call it revolution?—our society has been passing through, particularly in the last decade.

Contemporary society has gradually demanded a structural renovation of both the grass roots and the top levels. This society has anxiously tried to achieve a stable balance where, without detriment to the respect to which the human being in entitled, the individual may replace the social—a substitution which should be envisaged both for a society made up of small groups, as in the case of the family, and for the larger communities, whether national or international.

A knowledge of all these facts becomes important when we endeavour to rehabilitate the disabled so as to integrate them in the society for the building-up of which they can and should contribute. As we all know this object should be attained as far as possible through a process of total rehabilitation, i.e. one which takes into consideration the disabled and all his remaining potential, all his problems—physical, mental, social, economic and professional.

Reprinted with permission from *Paraplegia, 16:* 206-11. Copyright © 1978, Longman Group Ltd.

It is undoubtedly true that the integration or reintegration of the spinal cord injury patient in the community comes up against serious problems in a world where he had to work and live with at least a minimum of dignity. Among present-day problems in our world and which affect every human being, including the paralysed, unemployment looms large as an addition or as a sequel to them.

In fact, if we take into account the great changes that have occurred in the world at large and that the training made available to a given person (be he disabled or not) at a time of swift change as our own is no longer obtained as in times past, we are forced to go further than the mere "training of persons for the functions they will discharge later" and be content with this. Even when this is so, at least to some extent, it should be borne in mind that, for instance, a young paraplegic will be trained for a profession which he may have to discharge from his 20th year of age until retirement—in other words, over a period of time that may be as much as 40 years. This time-span is too long if we consider the ever greater advances of science and knowledge and their practical consequences. Thirty years ago no one would imagine that it would be possible to teach computer science in a school. And a little over 30 years ago no one could foresee the appearance of professions having to do with the exploitation of nuclear energy. No doubt that in a world in continuing change, what is particularly important is not so much to become adjusted, as the capacity for adjustment.

This is the reason why—apart from all that is basic and imminent in human nature and in the formation of the human person for a full discharge of the rights and duties—all the rest in teaching should be oriented towards a natural form of activity in evolution. "It is possible," says Leprince-Ringuet "to foresee accurately short-term techniques, say 5 years from now, but it is already highly uncertain when we look ahead 10 years whether in the field of technology proper or as regards the number of technicians. Beyond 10 or 15 years there is every probability of falling into error rather than otherwise." Thus, when considering teaching or technical training programmes for the disabled in vocational training centres, or outside them, we should take these facts into account and try to avoid detrimental routines, undergo

retraining from time to time in the form of more or less prolonged
on-the-job training periods so as to bring our knowledge up to
date, or eventually opt for a change in profession if circumstances
render this advisable.

In connection with what was mentioned before, another
important factor to take into consideration by all those engaged
in the rehabilitation of the spinal cord injury patient, is the
impact of environment and personality on disability. It is felt
already during the process of medical and vocational rehabilitation but doubtlessly more so in the case of reintegration in the
family, a job, or society generally. Man's ability to sustain himself
as an independent individual on the basis of work, in spite of the
impact an injury may have had in reducing or apparently
destroying it, is often determined in the interplay between
personality, environment and *disease.* However, the results
obtained through exhaustive investigation, carried out by Dr.
Gudmund Harlem (1974), seem to confirm that disease—even
when chronic—is not the most important nor determinant of
these factors. "Impairments and social problems are connected"
but it is not yet sufficiently clear what establishes this connection—a very important element to assess.

COUNSELLING THE DISABLED

In the entire process of rehabilitation of the disabled and with a
view to their more efficient integration to the community,
counselling plays an eminent role in the team work.

Team work, as Joseph Stubbins (1967) rightly points out,
"then becomes an interacting partnership or profession dealing
with the fundamental needs of the patient as a whole person." To
divide knowledge into separate fields is a matter of convenience.
In fact there is a considerable amount of overlap. This overlapping of activities of the various members of a rehabilitation
team should, however, contribute to stress or enhance the specific
work of each team member and not, of course, to replace it. And it
sould be advisable for this to be so even when the criteria are not
exactly the same. Mutual respect for other members of the team,
plus an overriding interest in the client and his problems, should
prevent differences of opinion from obstructing the team goal of
optimum rehabilitation of the client.

In counselling the client, the objects to be attained are as a rule restricted, the focus being namely on the elimination of incapacitating symptoms or negative attitudes, though the counselor will not cease trying to bring out and develop all the client's remaining potential. Non-acceptance of the disability, lack of cooperation of the client in one or another aspect of the prescribed rehabilitation programme, lack of will-power or motivation in starting the vocational training, and the desire to remain dependent on his relatives, are instances of frequent situations.

Nevertheless, the importance should be stressed of establishing limits of action in counselling the client. Both the counsellor and the patient should bear in mind that life cannot usually be changed. All one can do is just to change our own way of facing life and its problems. A good number of severely disabled clients, in fact, carry along with them complex problems which only indirectly have a bearing on the disability, or even have nothing whatever to do with it.

In any case the counsellor's help, though difficult, is indispensable to make it easier for the client to return to a productive type of life. This help is particularly necessary when a client's disability has a relation with his capacity for work which is not understood. "The most difficult part of the counsellor's job is the achievement of permanent employment for his patient and in getting civic leaders' and businessmen's attention and cooperation to create job opportunities for the disabled." We have here a challenge to the competence and dynamism of the counsellor in counselling not only the client, but also, quite often, the employers as well. This and other reasons should also stress the need for follow-up, that is "keeping in contact with the patient once the agency services are over."

COMMUNICATION IN COUNSELLING THE DISABLED

Any hospital or rehabilitation centre is to a large extent judged through its staff, that is, through their professional competence and their possibilities of human contact. And in accordance with Stubbins, "good teamwork requires good communication, not just reporting to the group and exchanging opinions. There is need for an awareness of the actions and interactions of the other professions with the patient, and a perceptiveness as to what observations will be useful to them. Team spirit, to which patients are extremely sensitive, is born of collaboration of all members of a competent team. If morale is high, it will be transmitted to the patient. It will spark in him the will to live and become proficient in living no matter what his handicap."

Herein lies the reason why the actions and objectives of human relations, through well-conducted communication, will be all the more successful the better the active co-operation between all those who collaborate in the organisation, including volunteers or even visitors.

Communication thus may become a basically important element or an excellent opportunity in counselling the patient. His reactions may, however, vary in accordance with the patient's age, temperament and/or mentality, and the type of injury. In this respect, Sir Ludwig Guttmann (1973) refers a very significant remark about the frame of mind of people meeting paraplegics: the case of a wounded priest—who wrote: "One of the most difficult tasks of a paraplegic is to cheer up his visitors." Often, it depends upon the manner of approach used by the doctor or any other member of the staff or visitors when communicating with the patient.

In fact the nature of communication will doubtlessly depend on information. This latter obviously suggests the idea of a transmitter which broadcasts in a more or less direct manner to a receiver. However, the idea of "transmission" leaves the phenomenon of communication incomplete. According to Albou, the fundamental expression is that of *reciprocity* or rather, of feedback: the individual is aware of the changes he produces in his interlocutor. His action is not executed independently of its effects, which are echoed or feedback the act of communication. Reciprocity and role alternation are thus the essential trait of communication.

In its turn, information will depend a great deal on the informer, his intellectual, moral and technical qualities, the latter being viewed from the standpoint both of professional competence and of an adequate knowledge of human relations.

Besides the members of the rehabilitation team, the informer may be the patient, or even the public in general.

Frequently the patient may ask more or less anxiously for information in order to integrate his experience and feelings into a reality he can understand so as to be able to cope with the new situation. Or, when asking for information, he may be expressing concern about his future and that of his family. If he is not listened to and understood, it is quite possible that he will ask himself whether those who deal with his rehabilitation are sufficiently competent to treat him. Hence the great responsibilities of the entire personnel dealing with the total rehabilitation of the spinal cord injury patient entrusted to their care, and in particular the doctor and the rehabilitation officer (or rehabilitation counsellor). "The counsellor," say Cull and Hutchinson (1975), "is not expected to know everything, but he is expected to develop a genuine relationship. As with the other qualities, a lack of genuineness or accuracy of responding will impair the counsellor's progress."

Verbal and nonverbal communication are of equal importance. From the tone of the counsellor's voice—which should be maintained at conversation level except when appropriately raised—the choice of words and the full attention given to the client instead of reading a folder, a report or a letter while the client is talking to the counsellor, a number of points should be carefully observed by the latter. Thus the counsellor must always control the interview because if he does not, if the roles played by the counsellor and the client were to be switched, counselling would cease. It is thus indispensable that throughout the interview the counsellor gives his best attitude of attention to the client, trying in the entire process of communication not only to listen to him, but also to hear and understand him. As Cull and Hutchinson (1975) quite rightly state, "in counselling there is a vast difference between listening and hearing. Hearing implies a greater degree of understanding of what is being said than listening implies. The counsellor should therefore be aware of what the client is communicating on a more basic meaningful level."

According to Elsa L. Ramsden (1975), the professional should not attend to only part of the speaker's message. When a patient talks he also sends non-verbal messages which help the listener interpret the real meaning of the message. For the patient may say in words "I feel okay," but this nonverbal behavior may indicate that, in fact, everything is not all right. This clarification of the patient's message may reveal to us the various objectives he is pursuing through his words. Ramsden cites in this connection an example which is current in rehabilitation centres. Consider, for instance, this patient's words: "Will I ever be able to walk again?" "The focus will be on *ever* with reference to time; or the focus may be on *walk* with the meaning related to the efficiency or normalcy of the walk." In order to answer the right question it is, of course, important to determine the real meaning, whether by a greater stress on each of the words *ever* or *walk* by the patient, or bearing in mind not only the contents of the sentence but also the feeling communicated. The "content" may be just a request for information about potential ability in ambulation, whereas the "feeling" may be an expression of anxiety or fear that, indeed, he will not be able to walk again.

The foregoing considerations allow us to foresee that successful counselling will depend a great deal on the ability to communicate. When learned and used with the highest and most balanced human interest, communication will undoubtedly be of the utmost value for better results in counselling the disabled.

SUMMARY

In the entire process of rehabilitation of the spinal cord injury patient, and with a view to a more efficient integration in the community, counselling plays an eminent role in the entire teamwork. Good counselling requires good communication. In its turn communication is based on appropriate information, and the latter will depend a great deal on the informer, both his professional competence and adequate knowledge of human relations. Only thus will it become possible to contribute to authenticity in psychological contacts, without which, whatever the means resorted to, there will be no true human communication and, therefore, the objective of counselling will not be attained.

REFERENCES

1. J. G. Cull and J. D. Hutchinson. Techniques of counseling in the

rehabilitation process. In J. G. Cull and R. E. Hardy (Eds.), *Vocational Rehabilitation Profession and Process*. Springfield: Thomas, 1975.

2. L. Guttmann, *Spinal Cord Injuries: Comprehensive Management and Research*. Oxford: Blackwell Scientific Publications, 1973.

3. G. Harlem, The impact of environment and personality on disability. *Internat Rehabil Rev*, Second Issue, 1973.

4. R. Hostie, *La communaute relation de personnes*. Paris: Desclee de Brouwer, 1976.

5. L. Leprince-Ringuet, *Science et Bonheur des hommes*. Paris: Flammarion, 1973.

6. A. Mehrarbian, *Silent Messages*. Belmond, CA: Wadsworth, 1971.

7. E. L. Ramsden, The patient's right to know—implications for interpersonal communication processes. *Physical Therapy Rev*, 55, 1975.

8. V. M. Santana Carlos, *Communication in Rehabilitation—A Contribution for Social Integration of the Disabled*. Paper presented at the International Federation on Public Relations in Rehabilitation, Athens, 1975.

9. M. Stewart, The only patient without a visitor—so she paid. *The Sunday [London] Express*, September 28, 1975.

10. J. Stubbins, El consejero entrenado profesionalmente aporta una nueva dimension a la rehabilitacion. *Revista Interamericana de Psicologia*, 1, 1967.

Chapter 13

ANTICIPATORY GRIEF, DEATH AND BEREAVEMENT: A CONTINUUM

AUSTIN H. KUTSCHER

I t has been said that there are two things that man cannot face—the sun and his own death. Yet, from the very instant of birth, we are on a long, it is *hoped*, trajectory toward death. Notwithstanding, all too few of us realize that a life is filled with major and minor preparations for death. There are constant *superficial* losses whose value in the process of this preparation should not be underestimated. The loss of a job, even voluntary movement from one job to another, loss of job seniority, loss of social status, loss of financial security, all are certain, less evident, examples of factors in this preparatory process. How many children survive their first haircut without tears? How many longhaired youth today dread, with accompanying and often extreme emotional conflicts, the parturition from this possession? And speaking of parturition, all are aware of the postpartum "blues," which often are seen to follow childbirth, and their sometimes devastating effects on many young mothers. All of these preparatory losses can be accompanied by and complicated by evidences of grief, both anticipatory, prior to the loss, and consequent, following the loss.

Therefore, it has been concluded by some, Dr. Arthur C. Carr[1] for instance, that these losses prepare the human being for the *greater* losses in his life, the deaths of his loved ones, and finally the loss of his own life. As caregivers in the economy of a human's

From Austin H. Kutscher, Anticipatory Grief, Death and Bereavement: A Continuum. In Kutscher, Austin H. and Goldberg, Michael R. (Eds.): *Caring for the Dying Patient and His Family: A Model for Medical Education,* 1973, pp. 11-23. Reprinted with permission of Health Sciences Publishing Corp., New York.

being, we should theorize about his ability to *accept* these losses through certain adaptive processes which include anticipatory grief and the work of bereavement; and we should try to affect the psychosocial consequences and patterns of his recovery from them at the same time that we also assist our dying patients to the boundaries of mortality. Death must be accepted and faced—the death of the individual and the death of the loved ones who predecease him.

When a fatal illness is diagnosed, as death approaches, and after the patient's death, there are many who are involved in the care of the patient as part of his trajectory: his family, the nurse who tends him, the physicians who treat his illness, and the minister and social worker, among others, who offer spiritual guidance and counsel. In addition to the dying patient, all of these important role players, some to a greater and others to a lesser extent, usually pass through stages of one or another form of grief and bereavement and/or deal with the emotional problems of terminal care by various defense mechanisms, such as denial. In trying to conceptualize this, the context of the title of this discourse is offered, to wit: the continuum of anticipatory grief, the dying of the patient, the death as experienced by survivors, and bereavement.

According to Dr. Elisabeth K. Ross, in her book *Death and Dying*,[2] the dying patient proceeds along a path characterized by various stages until as the optimum, he is enabled to achieve the point, or stage, of acceptance. These stages are 1) denial and isolation—failure to acknowledge the facts, disbelief in the face of overwhelming medical evidence, and a compulsion to be alone—to isolate himself, submerged in the depths of depressed and anxious thoughts; 2) anger—it can't be true, someone is lying, the doctors don't know what they are doing; 3) bargaining—if I do this, it won't be so; if I do that, perhaps something heroic, there will be a postponement of what seems to be inevitable: 4) depression—the sense of great loss; the reduction of the self-image; the realization of one's own shattered mortality and vulnerability; stress over the impact of medical expenses that go on and on; worry over the family at home; the realization that soon all will be lost, that the "me" will be gone from the scene; that death must be faced—and finally, if it can be reached, stage 5) acceptance—the inevitable will come no matter what is done; it must be faced by "me"; all will be lost; I do not know what will follow, but so be it: I have lived my life and tried to do my best.

Grief is the phenomenon of human behavior in survivors which accompanies loss; and its most striking effects are apparent when a beloved figure departs from life. The classic study of grief reactions was written by Dr. Erich Lindemann,[3] now himself critically ill, who observed and treated both the victims and their survivors following the tragic Coconut Grove nightclub fire that took place in Boston in the 1940's. According to Lindemann, grief is a definite syndrome with somatic and psychological symptomatology, although medical definition may not recognize it as such. The most striking characteristics are weeping, a tendency to sighing respiration, complaints about lack of strength, feelings of physical exhaustion, digestive disturbances (such as inability to eat, repugnance toward food and/or abdominal discomfort), etc. The bereaved may demonstrate a sense of unreality and detachment and may be intensely preoccupied with the image of the departed one. Guilt concerning acts done or not done may plague him; accompanying this guilt are extreme feelings of irritability and anger expressed towards others or toward the deceased. The bereaved person is frequently restless but unable to initiate meaningful activity. Even in the performance of his daily routine, he finds the smallest effort almost beyond his energies and capabilities. Depression, agitation and insomnia aggravate his physical and mental status.

Frequently, however, grief may have found its fullest expression before the death of this loved person. Its effects strike the bereaved-to-be at the moment the hopeless prognosis is pronounced, as he becomes aware of the truth of the situation. Therefore, the process of mourning can begin before the significant loss. It is contended here that during this period of anticipatory grief, the bereaved-to-be passes through some parallel, if not identical or synchronous, stages in relation to the dying patient (stages which would be positively identifiable if accorded similar and adequate study): He denies and disbelieves the medical evidence; he isolates himself, fearing that a sharing of his thoughts and doubts will only aggravate his torment and that of the dying patient and other members of the family. He is angry—perhaps at the patient who "hadn't taken care of himself" and who is going to leave him to face the world alone—perhaps also to raise a family alone; or, maybe at the doctors who refuse to do enough, or who are incapable of doing enough, or who may, he thinks, be lying to him or who are inordinately brutal in disclosing the facts; or, perhaps at the nurse who brushes aside his agonizing questions because it is not in her province to answer them, or who is agonized herself by them and shields herself by denial, or who never seems to be around when she is needed, or who seems to be adding to the patient's discomfort when she fails to respond immediately to his ring—for, very likely the same reasons; or perhaps at God;—or perhaps at various combinations of these people and a host of others.

The family member, in this context almost always a spouse or a parent, begins to bargain—if I do this, maybe pain will disappear, maybe even my loved one will be healed; if only I pray hard enough; if I perform some other demanding effort, this misery will go away and life will continue as before. He becomes depressed by thoughts of the present, by facts and fantasies of what the future will bring in suffering for all concerned—both during and after the course of the illness; he finds that he cannot function, cannot summon up either his emotional or physical resources to face each day as it comes; and so he is anxious, depressed and grieves—even mourns. Finally, hopefully, he accepts the facts: death will come; it must and will be faced; and I will be left to do as best I can in the future; there is no choice, and I must do what has to be done. —And, eventually, I too will face my own mortality: will I, and how will I, be able to accept that.

There appears to be a timetable of grief, oriented to both the date of the onset of a fatal illness as well as to the date of the loved one's death. And this timetable relates the period of grief to an undetermined but finite period of time. The presence of grief in anticipation of the loss, in both subtle and in pronounced ways, alters the trauma of the aftermath. When death has been prepared for by those who will survive, these bereaved may more readily find their way back to normal functioning. The contention here, requiring intensive study, is that there is a kind of symmetry and replication of effects: the more the anticipatory grief reaction before the loss, the less the bereavement effects following it: the less the anticipatory grief reaction before the loss (as must be inevitable in cases of sudden accidental death or death from an acute myocardial infarction or heart attack) the more the bereavement effects after the loss. Anticipatory grief creates an atmosphere, however ineffable, of adjustment to the potential loss; and so, to continue our hypothesis, then, is not anticipatory grief in its most simplistic course and form, a generally repressed projection backward of bereavement itself?

The physical symptomatology of grief is most apparent during the bereavement period. The bereaved person presents with a multitude of symptoms, as Lindemann and more recently Dr. Paula Clayton,[4] have related. Further and extensive studies, by Dr. Dewi Rees in Wales, Dr. C. Murray Parkes in England and Dr. David Maddison in Australia, have also produced data which indicate a greatly and clinically significantly higher morbidity rate among the bereaved (particularly following the loss of a spouse and especially in the older age groups) and, more importantly even, a higher rate of mortality during the first 6 months of bereavement—tapering off thereafter. Neglect of the self, for instance, may play some part, but there are some disease processes that cannot truly be related in such a manner, among them perhaps even cancer. It is contended here that parallel studies of anticipatory grief would likely reveal comparable findings.

Emotionally, both the patient's attitudes and desires and those of the bereaved-to-be may change from day to day: now he may want to hear the truth and talk about it; tomorrow he may detach himself from it and/or deny it—depending on the stage a-chieved—and the changes of patient and family may or may not be synchronous. Not at all unrelated to the above, a new fact or sign or happening—and interactions to this—may occur, partic-ularly within the cold walls of the institutional setting, with complicated emotional outcomes for all involved.

It is documented fact that most people today, in this country, die in hospitals and not at home (as was more often the case in the past). The hospital represents scientific achievement, the hope for cure with new and remarkable medications or machines, or, at least, a dream of prolonging the life of a beloved one. But hospitalization in itself causes separation; separation results in anxiety; separation anxiety in turn further reduces the contact of both family and friends with the patient, and, by so doing, increases everyone's anticipatory grief reaction; and the dying person, detached from his familiar surroundings and unable to be a vital member of society, goes through this period in a most extreme state of anxiety, suffering his own highly specific form of separation anxiety and anticipatory grief.

The patient may have complaints, but they frequently mask what his *real* complaints are—among many others, fear of death, distrust of those who, he often rightfully feels, may be concealing facts or at least something from him, and so forth. He truly has the right to grieve his own dying but is seldom given the opportunity to express his feelings and concerns. He usually finds himself being abandoned as his condition deteriorates; the living have already "written him off." He becomes the central figure in a great "conspiracy of silence"—forbidden to voice his fears and lied to concerning his condition and prognosis. The dying patient nearly always knows the truth but often doesn't know whether his kin have actually been told the worst. In the process, he may become antagonistic to them or, in many cases, may try to protect and shield his loved ones from the knowledge that he has. And this brings us to that widely debated question: Should the patient be told the truth, that death for him is imminent?

Although we have been debating this subject for decades, from the above it may be surmised that I think that this may actually be the wrong question. The question to be coped with should really be: How should we deal with what we must assuredly assume he "knows" or has discerned?—what Reverend Robert Reeves[5] describes as the "moment of truth" between the patient and his bereaved-to-be.

First of all, let it be understood that the nurse often talks the most with the patient and is in the best position to "read his signals." Her counsel should always be considered as extremely relevant. The life-style of the patient should be considered—how he handles trouble, reacts to bad news, responds in a crisis. And the life-style of the person in attendance who does the "telling"— the doctor, family member, or pastor—is also a factor which will profoundly affect the patient's future relationships with all those about him. And let us not forget that these caregivers who themselves are often desperately anxious about death including their own, whether consciously or unconsciously, may convince themselves erroneously through denial mechanisms that the patient does not know the truth—nor does he want to.

Most patients actually seem to fear the process of dying more than the unknown quantity, death. Yet, if those who will mourn his death would share their feelings with him in the living *now*, if emotional *expression* rather than emotional *repression* were to be allowed, many fears could be allayed and, for many more, the terminal days could be a time for a kind of exquisite loving, sharing and planning; and anticipatory grief for all would take on its most useful form and beneficent qualities. When there has been a free exchange of thoughts and emotions between two married people, or parents and a child under these circumstances, the survivor is left with a substantial foundation on which to rebuild his life—a product of the positive effects of anticipatory grief—and, with memories which become supportive during the days of sorrow and bereavement which follow the death. All such experiences represent a catharisis that ultimately allows the one to accept his own death with less fear (because he knows that he is loved and will not be abandoned) and his survivors to face the future with greater strength and a more suitably adjusted and positive life pattern. Hence, let us recapitulate the continuum of anticipatory grief, dying and bereavement, well or badly enacted, as suggested in the title of this essay.

Too often the caregivers delude themselves into what I called above "the conspiracy of silence." The terminal patient is shielded from the truth. True, not all patients do want to know and not all should necessarily be told; and if denial of the truth is the *only* way a patient can handle his dying, then he *should* be allowed his denial. But the greatest cruelty is inflicted when the patient *does* want to know and is *not* told. Observation has revealed that most patients crave an opportunity to ventilate their thoughts and feelings. Only in recent years, however, through the work of Dr. Herman Feifel, Dr. Elisabeth Ross and Dr. Avery Weisman, among others in the field of psychiatry and psychology, has the value of allowing the dying patient to ventilate his fears been appreciated. Perhaps above all, though, both for the patient and for his family, hope should never be utterly destroyed. The treatment plan should always be projected beyond the presumed life expectancy, recent conceivably hope-engendering developments in medical research can be discussed, etc.—so that at least a glimmer of hope never dies. And even when hope for survival is only a very dim and fading light indeed, a whole new series of realistic, achievable goals can effectively be introduced for all involved so that life may be lived to the very end. Such realistic goals can be, for example, strong reinforcement of the already acknowledged and existent love of a spouse, the summoning of strength to live until a grandchild is born, the settling of unsettled and hence troubling personal affairs, the resolution of family difficulties and intensively personal differences between the dying patient and surviving members of the family; reconciliations; and perhaps most important of all, in some instances, the hope of achieving what Dr. Ross has called "acceptance"—in the wake of which death with dignity can then be achieved.

In Great Britain, Dr. Cicely Saunders has established a "resting place for the weary traveler," the dying person, called St. Christopher's Hospice, a unique—and I should not perhaps, since she does not, even call it this—hospital for the terminally ill, where heroic measures are not taken to sustain life or prolong dying, where pain is controlled even as it starts, where dying truly becomes a part of living as the very walls of the hospital are breached to allow the family to enter at will; where a staff of compassionate and unbelievingly dedicated, in some instances highly religiously dedicated as well, people has been enlisted to support and tend the patient and permit him to die in dignity.

Such professionals, our caregivers, both on the scene and behind the scenes, are involved not only in their professional capacities but also personally and emotionally—with anticipatory grief and, thereafter, to some degree or other, with actual bereavement. How many—or, perhaps, we should ask, how few—nurses and physicians don't reach a point of emotional overload during periods when it seems that one patient after another dies in spite of all their combined and/or individual efforts to save or extend a life? And so, by way of answer, we pose some further queries—Why do some professionals avoid service

in wards where terminal patients are moved to die? Why do so
many others tend to abandon the patient as his condition
deteriorates, to visit him less frequently, to perform only those
acts which treat his primary illness, to hustle and bustle in and
out of the room as rapidly as possible, avoiding conversation
which may prove to be embarrassing and to avoid answering
questions, fearful that their own acknowledgment of the patient's
psychological distress, *and their own,* will bring forth tears—
maybe even their own? Somehow or other, incidentally, we
regard crying in ourselves and others as unworthy, unmanly or as
an inappropriate reaction—when such is *not* the case at all.

I would like at this point to offer some succinctly expressed
words to serve, it is my hope, as a few effective tools, many set
forth by Avery Weismann,[6] for all who care for the dying patient
and his family.

1. The caregiver's chief obligation is to provide what Weisman has so imaginatively called "safe conduct" for the dying
patient.

2. The primary suffering of the patient is handled by those
who can relieve the physical symptoms of his ailment, especially
his pain or his disfigurement; but his secondary sufferings—the
lost of self-esteem and body image, the fears of abandonment and
separation, the anxieties and feelings of hopelessness, must also
be treated...by *anyone* who can function well in this capacity.

3. The reactions of particularly close family members should
be scrutinized in order to help them and to enable them, those
who are losing the most, to do the most to relieve the patient's
secondary suffering; and in so doing gain a measure of peace
themselves.

4. High risk family members, those adjudged to be most
prone to suffer at some point from pathological and extended
grief reactions following their loss, should be singled out for
special counselling and treatment.

5. The patient should be allowed to make as many decisions
regarding his own treatment, even his own manner of dying, as is
consistent with *his* welfare, not heeding needlessly only the
emotional welfare of his family or especially that of his *caregivers.*

6. Communication should always be maintained among all
on the scene; self-esteem should be reinforced.

7. There are many, including especially family members, who can help the dying patient achieve his final goals—not only the physician and the nurse. Professional credentials are oftentimes less important than a person's ability to be present, to be readily available, to be alert, to be compassionate and willing to be on the team. And, touch the patient; let there be someone to hold his hand, literally, if possible, to the end.

8. The team should include, among others, the family, the clergy, social workers, psychologists and psychiatrists as well as physicians and nurses.

9. The new ethics, presented by the ability to transplant organs or sustain failing ones mechanically, compel the physician to be the prime decision-maker, the one in whose hands the "buck stops." But, nevertheless, these decisions and ethics involved pose profound and emotionally traumatic problems for the physician which he would be well advised to share with the family, clergy or others.

10. The family should always be aware that to the physician, regardless of his concerns about the patient, one death in particular is of even greater concern to him: his own death.

11. The bereaved will have to deal retrospectively with the trauma of the deceased's illness and death and he may be haunted by memories, even guilt and anger. Caregivers must be available to contend with these also.

12. The passing on of certain cultural and ethnic rituals, such as portions (at least) of formal funerals, sitting shiva, and the wake, has probably been detrimental for the family as viewed sociologically and can hinder acceptance of the loss and the bereaved's ability to continue as a functioning human being. These rites and the attendant opportunities for loving companionship and self-expression often offer great emotional support to the bereaved—even if many do not choose to acknowledge such benefits because of not infrequently unfair financial burdens imposed by some funeral directors.

13. The grief experience can be transformed into a most meaningful and productive one through emphasis of the concepts and ideals of *creative* grief. The energies expended in grieving can be channeled with enormous productivity into good works or deeds, service to others in distress, devotion to tasks left

undone by the deceased, etc., rather than dissipated in an unstructured, self-pitying melancholia.

But all of the answers are not here. We have scarcely scratched the surface. Even the few statistics drawn upon may be viewed dubiously because we are just beginning to gain insight into *what* to research, and such research efforts have just barely been started. One more observation is in order. Our efforts in this field may need reappraisal since it appears that for every 15 investigators working in giving care to the dying patient, there are probably only three dealing with bereavement, and only one with studies of anticipatory grief. This is discouraging to relate, in the opinion of many of our most informed workers in the field of thanatology, since the possibility for the most effective interventive medical action related to bereavement perhaps lies in the improved management of anticipatory grief.

We have turned around and around in our continuum: the classical picture of anticipatory grief, the dying experience and its management, and the final facet, bereavement. Nor have we neglected to mention our own psychological trauma at the thought of the dying "me." It should be apparent, then, that we have come full cycle and have, perhaps, even reached certain conclusions:

1) That our lives *are* spent in preparation for the bereavement which our great losses bring, including the death of "me"; 2) that there are doubtlessly stages of anticipatory grief which in one way or another parallel Dr. Ross's stages of dying—in a complementary fashion, sometimes and best of all in synchronization but sometimes out; 3) that, if we can achieve some degree of real synchronization, we can make the bereaved-to-be function more satisfactorily as members of the team that cares for the terminal patient; 4) that the mortality and morbidity of bereavement may well, with proper research and through the use of proper investigative expertise, be demonstrated in anticipatory grief, thereby reinforcing the decision to intervene at this point; 5) that it is logical to conceive of anticipatory grief as a repressed projection backward of bereavement; 6) that it would follow, then, that bereavement is the logical aftermath of repressed anticipatory grief; 7) that there is a symmetry and core of replication between anticipatory grief and bereavement from which it might

well be hypothesized that the greater and better managed the one, the less of the other; and conversely, the less of the former, the greater the latter; 8) that these are challenging and critical areas for research.

Man cannot face the sun, but he must nevertheless face his own death, if he is to live. He must accept death as a part of his life—as a prerequisite for his enjoyment of and formal acceptance of the full beauty and tragedy of life. Just as it is possible for the dying person to achieve acceptance of his own death and die in dignity, so too the living who are bereaved can, with help, be brought to accept a life in which death is an integral part. The challenge to us all is at least twofold: where is our place in the continuum at any time? how can we be effective as clinicians, as scientists and as humane beings?

REFERENCES

1. Arthur C. Carr, A lifetime of preparation for bereavement. In A. H. Kutscher (Ed.), *But Not to Lose*. New York: Frederick Fell, 1969.
2. Elisabeth Kubler-Ross, *Death and Dying*. New York: Macmillan, 1969.
3. Erich Lindemann, Symptomatology and management of acute grief. *Am J Psychiatry, 101:*141, 1944.
4. Paula J. Clayton, Evidences of normal grief. In A. H. Kutscher (Ed.), *Death and Bereavement*. Springfield, Thomas, 1969.
5. Robert B. Reeves, Jr., The hospital chaplain looks at grief. In B. Schoenberg, A. C. Carr, D. Peretz, and A. H. Kutscher (Eds.), *Loss and Grief; Psychosocial Management in Medical Practice*. New York: Columbia University Press, 1970.
6. Avery Weisman, Psychosocial considerations in terminal care. In Schoenberg et al., *op. cit.*

Chapter 14

SPECIALTY ROUNDS: PSYCHOSOCIAL ROLES IN THE CANCER DRAMA

NATHAN SCHNAPER, ANNE P. HAHN AND RACHEL DEVRIES

All the world's a stage,
And all the men and women merely players;
They have their exits and their entrances;
(Jacques) Shakespeare, *As You Like It,*
Act II, Scene VII, Line 139

Life's but a walking shadow; a poor player,
That struts and frets his hour on the stage,
And then is heard no more;
(Macbeth) Shakespeare, *Macbeth,* Act V,
Scene V, Line 25

Any illness, particularly a life-threatening one, has an aura of drama for the patient—the labile emotion, the conflict and, unfortunately, the oppressive suspense. The verses from Shakespeare reflect somewhat pessimistically the ambiance of the cancer drama. Certainly, life has a temporal quality, but need not be hopeless or desperate. This fact will become evident by the three cases we are presenting at these specialty rounds.

Cancer is a life-threatening disease, as are fulminating and nonfulminating cardiovascular, renal, neurologic, pulmonary, and other systemic illnesses. However, the "patient with cancer"

Reprinted with permission from *The American Journal of Medical Sciences, 140:* 795-6. Copyright© 1978 by Charles B. Slack, Inc.

serves well as a model for discussion of the emotional concomitants of life-threatening illnesses. While there are general considerations applicable to the child as well as the adult, a formal discussion of the child with cancer is omitted. The management of the child and his/her family are important topics, but space limitations preclude the lengthy attention they merit.

Subtle psychological concepts exert a powerful influence on all the actors in this life-threatening drama. They are (1) the unconscious, (2) transference, and (3) defenses.[1] One sees *the unconscious* revealed in dreams, slips of the tongue and pen, hypnosis, and emotional symptoms. There are things we can tell our closest confidantes (secrets), things we can only tell ourselves (fantasies), and things that we cannot tell even ourselves (out of our awareness-unconscious). The unconscious has little regard for reality and is timeless. The more likely that an experience is painful or shameful, the more likely it will be repressed into the unconscious. This powerful source can determine an individual's behavior, compelling him to act in ways seemingly irrational to the current situation.

Transference is also unconscious and impels one to respond emotionally to important people as one did to father, mother, and other significant persons in one's childhood. This phenomenon has ramifications in the patient-provider relationship.

Physical and physiological *defenses* are well known, but there are also emotional defenses against anxieties in one's inner and outer environment. In a situation where one experiences conflict or threat of personal injury or loss, or threat of loss of love, security, or self-esteem, anxiety signals the defensive process. The defenses can be utilized constructively or destructively, and begin in earliest childhood and develop experientially.

A few of the defense mechanisms relevant to the participants in the cancer drama are:
1. *Repression:* unconscious forgetting.
2. *Suppression:* conscious forgetting, eg, "I'll think about it tomorrow." But "tomorrow" comes too soon, proving the ineffectiveness of this defense.
3. *Denial:* which is unconscious, prevents one from seeing that which is unpleasant, particularly about oneself. This defense can spare one pain and preserve hope, as in the case

of a terminal illness. Conversely, denial can be used pathologically by patients who delay diagnosis and treatment.

4. *Displacement:* a defense whereby the emotion remains the same, although now unconsciously transferred to less anxiety provoking objects. The child who experiences a mask thrust upon his face, retaliates not to the anesthesiologist, but to a sibling or playmate.

5. *Projection:* a mechanism by which one's true feelings are unconsciously attributed to another. The patient may fear the side effects of chemotherapy and, thus, resent the oncologist. In time, he wonders if these noxious reactions are necessary or if they are deliberate punitive acts on the part of the oncologist, "who doesn't like me."

6. *Isolation:* the de-emotionalizing of an effect. Intellectualization is frequently utilized in the service of isolation. An example: discussing all aspects of one's cancer and its treatment as if one were talking about another patient.

Three cases will be described. The roles of the participants will be discussed separately. This separation is artificial, as interaction is constant, and is done only for purposes of clarity of presentaiton.

CASE REPORTS

Patient No. 1

A brilliant scientist died at age 46 of a melanoma. He was highly trained in the use of intellectual processes and at the same time, given to macho (masculine-virile) endeavors, eg, flying, mountain climbing, skiing, scuba diving. Despite vigorous therapy, including chemotherapy and several surgical procedures (axillary dissection, occipital lobe resection), he continued his intellectual and physical pursuits. To himself, he would not be "defeated by a melanoma" and to observers, he appeared to be successful. He, too, believed this, for in his case, macho equaled denial.

However, his wife's perceptions were not in concurrence with his. His personality changed, he was quieter, at times withdrawn or irritable. He tried to maintain the "macho image" to the end. He flew, he climbed mountains, and worked productively. A few days before he died, he attempted intercourse, but was too weak. His wife tried to reassure him that "it is not important to me," and his macho reply was, "but it is important to me!"

Patient No. 2

A young, attractive woman in her early 30s relapsed after a seven-year remission from Hodgkin's disease. It was not a simple process. For some time, she complained of backaches, but was reassured by her physicians that these were "only housewifely complaints." She sought relief by buying a new mattress, sleeping on the floor, etc. to no avail. Finally, her gynecologist ordered an intravenous pyelogram and it soon became evident that a tumor was impinging on her right kidney. Active therapy was then instituted.

This experience compounded a previously similar one. When first diagnosed, she and her husband were given little information and even told not to tell anyone the diagnosis. She was treated as a child, at times given instructions resembling "baby talk" (she possesses two academic degrees).

These two experiences, both occurring with awareness of illness, were available to her defensively. She became angry and bitter, but never verbally expressed these feelings to her doctors and ancillary personnel, and at the same time, denying that it was directed at her illness. Anger was deflected toward her husband in that she felt he was not "answering my questions" and not being responsive to her needs. She found it difficult to believe that her husband would not counter the anger with anger out of deference to her illness. Both confessed to not admitting their anger toward their providers. They feared retaliation in terms of the staff withholding part or all of therapy. "We depend on them. We are in their hands."

Patient No. 3

A woman in her 40s in remission from Hodgkin's disease was a talented artist who drew humorous cartoons as a running diary of her experiences from time of diagnosis through the present. She was popular with the staff, who found her likable but at the same time, were not cognizant of her anger and frustrations. Physicians, nurses, and therapies were portrayed in caricature. Doctors reflect their fallibility, the nurses' caps have devil-like horns, the treatments belittled to absurdity, and the captions a subtle sting cloaked in humor which served as a vehicle of expression for her anger.

Sexual innuendo was evident in almost all the cartoons. The exceptions were significant. During the many complications of her illness, the patient was portrayed as a voluptuous, sexy, scantily clad female. When symptom-free, the female was somewhat plain and clothed decorously.

At one particular period when she was asymptomatic, she drew nonsexual cartoons as usual, but suddenly, while still presumed by patient and staff to be asymptomatic, her cartoons took on an erotic coloring. Soon thereafter, she became symptomatic (a severe thoracic outlet syndrome). Her art work had expressed the body image changes that were occurring outside of her or the staff's conscious awareness.

These cases reflect the major characters poised at center stage in the cancer drama: the patient and his family. But there are other performers as well. Waiting in the wings are the supporting cast, the providers: the physicians, nurses, social workers, psychiatric consultants, and the nonmedical staff (in and out of the hospital). Responses of each are predicated on personality and previous experience.

THE PATIENT'S ROLE

Cancer! Despite advertisements and exhortations to reassure the public, the word still conjures up an immediate image of death and futility. For some people this evokes prompt and necessary action; in others, emotional paralysis, delay, and/or rumination. In either case, the defenses enumerated above are called forth. They are used singly or in various combinations to cope with the onslaught of anxiety. At this time, the anxiety is experienced as a stress with little or no possibility of resolution.

The anxiety is not limited to the fear of a "lingering, painful death," but has its roots in other sources. Finesinger, Abrams, Cobb, and Shands have thoroughly studied the problem of anxiety in cancer patients. In one study, 93% of the patients experienced guilt.[2,3] In another study, two thirds of the patients felt "it's my fault," "I've done something wrong."[4] ("Sins": sexual, eg, masturbation, and/or hostile aggression, eg, resentments of parents.) Other patients feel inferior or inadequate.

There are anxieties emanating from the fear related to death itself and its searching questions. For example, there is the fear of the unknown: "Will I rot after I am buried?" "Is there a Judgment Day?"[5] Also, there are fears centered on losses: of being separated from nurturing people who will be missed; the loss of body image, "Will I become emaciated?" "Will I smell bad?", the loss of control, "Will I reveal secrets as I weaken?" "Will I not have any say in what is done with my body while I'm still alive?"

Regression is also feared as it implies role reversal and dependency. As alluded to earlier, it can be a useful defense mechanism in that it permits cooperation with therapy. But there are those who resist it completely—refusing to participate in their treatment, rejecting all help. And there are those who capitulate to the defense by over-dependency, becoming child-like in their clinging and, at the same time, resenting the dependency.

Ongoing, from diagnosis to loss of consciousness or demise, grieving in one form or another takes place (*Vide infra*, Role of the Family: Grief).

The most effective defense against the reality of death is *denial*, either outright or indirect. Denial can manifest itself in many ways. This brings us to the actors in the three cases cited above, all of whom utilized denial in a "constructive way."

Patient No. 1

Machismo was this patient's technique for denial. Supporting his denial was his highly honed capacity for intellectualization. As a scientist, he functioned on an intellectual level. He discussed his "case" with great facility. By intellectualizing about his disease he obscured its reality and treated it as if it were another's clinical history. Like many patients with cancer, he could speak of his symptoms, the prognosis, the blood counts and related data, but only as a subject somehow apart from him. His denial was apparent in the following example: his wife wanted to bring his comfortable office chair home the week before he died. At that time, return to work was precluded by his physical incapacitation. He demured at the suggestion, saying "What will I do for a chair in my office?"

In the same idiom, he considered how he would terminate his life if he became incapacitated and no longer in control. He discussed with his wife overdosing on narcotics. However, when the time for decision came, he postponed action for a day. The next day he died naturally and quietly.

Patient No. 2

This bright young housewife denied any feelings of anger related to her Hodgkin's disease. Instead, she complained about, but not to, all doctors and ancillary personnel who crossed her path as she relapsed. Her denunciation of them was bitter and vehement. Her husband was the sole recipient of her anger. When questioned as to the degree of her anger (not *why* she was angry), she would shout, "I'm not angry about my illness, if that's what you're asking. I'm angry with everybody's stupidity!"

Anger for this patient reflected not a denial of relapse, but a denial of the possibility of hopelessness. She was "fighting mad" and hope was on her side. Because the anger was displaced, the staff was usually oblivious to its presence, a result, perhaps, of a need on the part of the staff to be liked.

When patients complain to others about their professional caretakers and are advised to tell the particular staff person how they feel, they refuse and, also, insist that the listener say nothing. Complaints are rare as they feel their survival is in the hands of the helpers. The fear is that any antagonism will kindle anger and the patient will be abandoned. When the patient is obsequious or overly deferential, underlying anger should be suspected. A simple comment to the patient such as, "I wonder if you're feeling fed up with all this business," could evoke verbalization.

Patient No. 3

Here denial is expressed, not as an intellectualization, not as anger, but as humor. This patient is laughing at herself—the cruel "joke" is on her. The reality of death has "lost its sting." Despite the humor in her cartoon captions, the edge of anger points toward her providers, but as with patient No. 2 the anger is never verbalized directly. In many of the cartoons, she is criticizing the language of the oncologists: the use of acronyms, protocols of therapy, techniques of bone marrow and lumbar punctures, radiotherapy, and technological advances in general.

The dynamics of portraying herself as provocative and volup-tuous during periods of symptomatic illness are of interest.

Certainly with active disease there are bodily changes. Could the sexy quality of her drawing be a denial of unpleasant body image changes?

As with all of us, these three actors have practiced their roles since childhood. Personalities do not "just happen," nor are they a result of an accident of fate. They develop gradually, and complexly, as a result of forces impinging from the individual's internal and external environments. Patterns of coping develop with experience. As people, patients respond to stress in ways they have always reacted to stress. Cancer is a stress. [6-10] The scientist, patient No. 1, used intellectualizations. Patient No. 2, who was always a kind of maverick, utilized anger to plead "Why me?" Patient No. 3 is an artist, and cartooning is her particular language style.

A phenomenon worthy of mention is the paradoxical response to "good news." Frequently, patients when told that their biopsy was negative or that they are now in a "solid" remission, will feel a great sense of elation followed by a period of depression. The suggested explanation is that these patients have their defenses (their "troops") always on the ready, only to find the effort no longer necessary. Also, they remain insecure, believing that "I'm OK now, but when will the axe fall? I have to sweat it out." One patient who had battled a breast cancer, recurrences, and metastases for six years, was told by an oncologist that with a "new" treatment, she "could be *cured*." After a day of high spirits, she became severely depressed. Her way of life had been geared to a total commitment of time and effort to fighting her cancer. Now she would no longer have anything to do and her life would be meaningless.

THE ROLE OF THE FAMILY

"Life is a passing shadow," says Scripture. The shadow of a tower or a tree? No: the shadow of a bird—for when a bird flies away, there is neither shadow nor bird.

Midrash: *Genesis Rabbah*, 80

Patients and their families interact with grief and mourning.[11-13] At times, separately and privately, and at other times, together and publicly, but at all times, each in their own way. Families play an integral part as the patients move through different phases of the disease. Their reactions directly and indirectly affect the patient and the helpers. They bring pressure on the providers to "spare" the patient and "not tell the truth." Implicit in this behavior is the guilt they feel for they themselves having been spared the disease. A common reaction is resentment toward the diagnosing doctor. This is intensified if the patient is a child. Anger is felt toward the "messenger" rather than the message.

What follows in the grief process applies equally to the patient and the survivors: the family's immediate response is shock and anguish, shared by the patient. *Why me?! Why him?! Why her?!* There are no answers to these questions, as no explanations, or known etiological factors are forthcoming. Nonetheless, patients and their families reach out with convincing explanatory fantasies: going out in the cold with wet hair; a neglected bee-sting; a fall from a horse; an unforgiving attitude; frequent masturbation, etc.

The initial shock response to the diagnosis introduces the *grief reaction* to the patient, his family, and friends. Death exacerbates the process for the survivors. Grief is the "normal" reaction to any loss or separation, eg, divorce, a financial catastrophe, loss of a job, graduation, aging. Grief "work" is a psychological necessity, a debt that must be paid.[14] The trauma must be assimilated and emotional ties severed. This must be resolved so that new relationships can be established. Mourning is manifest through the expression of the pain of grief.

There are overlapping phases to the grief reaction which can proceed progressively or skip or be pathologically delayed, chronic, or omitted. Following shock there is emotional release, usually tears. Emotion has been suspended and now the full impact of realization of the loss occurs. Fears are usual. Covert hostility is implicit in the protestations surfacing again as "Why?!" Why?! Why me?! Why him?! Why her?! (At times one hears the "Why me?!" from a family member suggesting anger toward the patient for "putting me through this.")

One observes the hopelessness, the loneliness, the helplessness, the sense of isolation, all combined under the rubric of utter depression. This period of depression can be the predominant one and can serve as painful expiation of guilt. Simultaneously, it can also, in a sense, provide a period of consolidation, an inventory of potential or actual loss again, shared by the patient and his family.

Other stages can follow, not necessarily in order: panic with difficulty in concentrating; anorexia and insomnia as well as more serious physical symptoms; overt expressions of guilt, with or without overt expressions of hostility toward the providers and/or family members; sadness at reminders of the potential loss or lost one; difficulty with usual activities; and, for the relatives after the patient's death, a gradual waning of grief and mourning over a period of weeks to two years and a readjustment to reality— one is "one's old self again." The above may be summarized as shock, turmoil, and resolution. Most patients and/or their families begin the grieving process at time of diagnosis. Other relatives delay until the death of the patient.

Morbid or pathological grief reactions can be manifested in foolish behavior, over-dependency, delayed or chronic grieving, litigenous behavior, suicidal attempts, and loss of the capacity to feel emotion of any kind. These reactions require the intervention of a psychotherapist, but need to be recognized by the helpers.

Fortunately, most families, as with many patients, cope with the crisis in a laudatory way. Some families, however, in an effort to obviate later feelings of guilt and loss, move too close to the patient and overwhelm him and the providers. Other families go to the opposite extreme and abandon the patient in order to protect themselves from the pain of the anticipated loss. Both techniques fail as the mourning process comes and is intense.[15]

With patients No. 1 and 2, their spouses mourned in their own ways, as expected. The wife of the scientist (patient No. 1) cried almost constantly during his illness but, since his death, only during the occasional reminders, eg, his aftershave odor in his clothes, a favorite song. The husband of patient No. 2 deals with his wife's illness (and anger) with an admission of, "I'm scared" and quietly accepts her shouting and almost anything that she demands of him. At times, though, he has to retreat into himself to "recharge his batteries."

It is incumbent upon the medical providers to be alert to the patient-family interaction. Thus, it becomes their function to simply observe, or intervene when necessary, steering the family to a middle ground. This serves the patient's and the family's best interests. The helpers must remain in the wings, off-stage and resist the impulse to suppress appropriate mourning by word or drug, intervening only when the process is pathological. The urge to suppress mourning of others stems from the need to allay one's own evoked anxiety.

It is generally assumed that the "professionals" working with the cancer patient include only the oncologist and the nurse. On a cancer unit the term includes the staff psychiatrist, clinical pharmacist, social worker, occupational and physical therapists, dietitian, and housekeeping personnel. Each contributes in his or her own way to the care of the patient. Essentially, they are providers, hopefully, helpers. At times, helpers with their own personality problems become strictly providers and no longer helpers. In the following presentation the clinical pharmacist, dietitian, occupational and physical therapists, and housekeeping providers will not be discussed. This does not imply any lack of significance on their part toward a fruitful team effort, as will be acknowledged in the section on Management.

THE ROLE OF THE PROFESSIONALS

The oncologist develops his personality in the same way as the patient. Indeed, when he himself is a patient, his utilization of defenses is similar to those of his patient—compounded by his role reversal. As physician-in-charge, he may have emotional conflicts which might be *displaced*, eg, anxieties in his marital relationship displaced onto his relationship with his patient or vice versa. Projection is played out when his omnipotence is threatened by his patient's imminent demise. In this situation, the doctor experiences the patient's actions as an attack on his training, competence, person, and the very integrity of his fantasies of being god-like. The doctor feels "up-staged."[16]

Patients do reinforce the doctor's fantasies by their magical expectations of him. So much so, that even though patients undergo painful procedures and are made to wait until what is felt a near eternity for the doctor, they will not complain because they feel their survival is in the doctor's hands. To the claim that the physician is dispassionate, they can counter that the doctor is busy (the defense of *rationalization:* an excuse that makes sense).

Also, that he must keep a "clinical distance," is an acceptable rationalization. At this point, the physician relinquishes his role as "helper" and is now simply a "provider."

The physician's feelings of omnipotence stem from the past.[15] The infant has the view that he is the center of the universe and, therefore, is indeed omnipotent. As he develops through a normal phase of ambivalence, he then becomes aware that there are others (mother, father, siblings) in his world. During this period he equates the wish with the deed. Should he wish someone to die (ie, "go away"), he is convinced this will happen. Simultaneously, he is frightened that should his wish be fulfilled, retribution will occur. The residue of this conflict persists in the doctor's unconscious, as it does with everybody. With awareness that his patient will die, he is compelled by unrealistic guilt and accountability to turn away, avoiding retaliation in kind. He unconsciously views his omnipotence as the ability to kill or cure. Unfortunately, this view can result in abandonment of the patient. It is fortunate that there are "healthy" doctors—those who have come to terms with their omnipotence. They stay in character and utilize their personality as is. If they are usually authoritative, they are so with their patients. If they like to jolly people along, they do so with their patients. In this way their approach is experienced by the patient as a sincere one.[16] The oncologist needs to have an awareness, not only of his patient's personality, but his own.[17] Thus, he can function with realistic pride in his skill, and can communicate this to the patient. He can then offer the patient information, assurance, reassurance, clarification, support, firmness when necessary, sympathy when indicated—each in an objective, reality-oriented way, and for mutual benefit.

There are significant differences in the role of the traditional liaison psychiatric consultant and that of the oncologic psychiatric consultant who spends half, or more, of his time on the cancer unit. The former "puts out fires," ie, patient consults on request of the primary physician, and generally is based outside the unit, or in some cases, outside the hospital. According to Lipowski, the "consultant is invariably a therapist."[18] He functions with staff as well as with patients. The oncologic psychiatric consultant who is willing to be involved will find his role as consultant increased. In time, he will be seen as a friend, counselor, partner, and even trouble-shooter and is asked "corridor consults" by staff members regarding patients, families, or themselves.

The oncologic psychiatric consultant performs the following functions simultaneously: as mediator between medical-biological and psychiatric-behavioral staff disciplines; consultant/therapist to patients at staff requests; consultant to other psychosocial staff; consultant to administrative staff as to policy relating to psychosocial management; researcher and teacher, holding individual or staff conferences; and educator to the lay community. While he does not practice "formal" or traditional psychotherapy in all cases, he does utilize brief supportive and/or confrontation psychotherapy. Psychotropic drugs are part of his armamentarium.

When the oncologic psychiatric consultant has the good fortune to be a member of the support structure to a research-oriented unit, his participation in research activities is unlimited. Psychosocial clinical problems abound—as the presentation of these rounds affirms. What specific coping techniques predominate? Do emotional problems influence recovery? Do premorbid psychosocial factors predispose to cancer? Can the psychosocial factors in patients, families and staff be quantitated? If so, by what instruments? and so on. At the Baltimore Cancer Research Center, there are presently collaborative studies of the psychological reactions of donors and recipients to transfusions of whole blood and cell components; body image perceptions and coping techniques in patients with recurrent breast cancer; effects of emotional trauma on the recovery rates of treated AKR mice.

There are satisfactions for the oncologic psychiatric consultant which include an appreciation and enhanced communication between the oncologic and psychiatric providers. Also, the oncologic psychiatric consultant has the rare opportunity to gain a perspective of medicine that complement his routine office practice. He can no longer separate the mind from the body as do some of his exclusively medical and purely psychiatric colleagues. Above all, there is the gratifying feeling of having a significant role to play in the cancer drama—a sense of belonging and being a team member coping with a serious disease.[19,20]

The cancer nurse is on line day in and day out and at times, must deal with patient and the family "on the spot."[21-24] The nurse is often left with the shocked or stunned patient and family who have many spoken and unspoken questions after being told by the doctor that the patient has cancer or that the leukemia has relapsed. The concerned nurse has the opportunity to make a meaningful contact with the patient while his defenses are at a low ebb. The nurse must develop a skill in handling "loaded" questions from patients. The seemingly straightforward questions are frequently checking out what the doctor has told the patient. It is tempting for the emotionally over-involved nurse to usurp the doctor's role. The nurse who relates openly and frankly with the patient and his family offers them education and predisposes them to deal more openly with others.

In the cancer setting, the social worker performs several roles. During various stages of the illness and subsequent adjustment process, the social worker may play a primary role dealing with emotional problems and conflicts besetting the family secondary to the disease. At other times, the social worker may assume a supporting role. This role could well be the one most utilized by a social worker in the hospital setting, and implies that the worker direct the family toward stability by referrals to appropriate resources or brief therapy. At other times in the course of the drama the social worker acts as a prompter. In this role she enhances and facilitates communication between the patient and family, family and physician, or within the cancer unit. [26-31]

The social worker's functions are not in conflict with those of the oncologic psychiatrist. Their work does overlap and is complementary. The social worker's services are implemented by patient and family interviews, patient or family meetings, and meetings with members of the health team, as well as lay groups. While traditional case work activity such as resource referral is performed, the oncologic social worker does more. There is interaction with the family, assisting them in identifying problems, and in making a reasonable plan for resolutions.

The emotional stress for the professionals merits some comment. The oncologic physician, nurse, social worker, and psychiatrist are subject to the "burned-out" phenomenon. Its implications are apparent. The constant exposure to dying and death with its painful twinges of failure of omnipotence predisposes to depression. For some this means a change of occupation. For others, a transient "down" followed by a renewed dedication. Friends and relatives of staff members find it difficult to understand how one can work on a cancer unit. And, it is difficult to explain why one does. Some conjectures as to motivation are: an intellectual denial of one's own mortality; an effort to master death by increased knowledge; a need to rework a personal loss; and possibly, a response to the challenge and thereby prove one's omnipotence. Not to be overlooked is the conviction that one is doing interesting and important work.

The day-to-day coping with the stress is subtle and unspoken— joking, teasing, and "one-liners" with each other. (This is common in the surgical operating room, and also for reasons of stress.) Group meetings are useful within each discipline, as are one-to-one meetings. Research provides clinical distance while nourishing a realistic sense of *partipotence* (partial omnipotence) at the same time. Outside activities and interests are crucial.

MANAGEMENT—ON STAGE EVERYONE

Sun Journey
Hope is like the sun,
which, as we journey toward it
casts the shadow of our burden behind us
                    Samuel Smiles, *The Eternal Light,* p. 130

It is assumed that all performers have learned their roles well and there is no longer an artificial separation of the various characters, but rather all interact with each other. The patient's physical and emotional well-being are intertwined, and his care therefore must include the whole range of patient-family provider reactions.

Simultaneously, there are patient-patient interactions contributing to the overall plot of the drama. These go on in the inpatient areas as well as in the outpatient waiting rooms. There are some who feel threatened by the remission of another patient. Others are threatened by another's relapse. And there are patients who form close relationships and others who keep their own company. All are very human reactions: resentment that another is "getting well, while I am not", or frightened that another is relapsing and, "am I next?"; closeness with other patients, sharing a common experience; or getting too close to many who soon die "and it hurts." (Obviously, interactions such as these are more apt to be played out in a cancer unit rather than in the office of the private physician.)

One useful therapeutic tool is the Patient Management Conference. It is held biweekly at the Baltimore Cancer Research Center and is multidisciplinary in orientation. The primary physician briefly presents the medical characteristics of the patient, the treatment, and the psychosocial problems(s). The senior associate follows with a discussion of the patient's particular protocol and its general implications. Input is then provided by the psychiatrist, social worker, nurses, dietitian, and anyone else who has knowledge about the patient or the problem(s). A consensus solution is then suggested. Problems include noncooperation with treatment, emotional decompensations, staff irritation, etc. The essential contribution of the conference is the presentation of a united front (mileu) to the patient by the staff, as well as the doctors and nurses viewing each other with respect, understanding, and cooperation.

The patient is coping with stress. He has cancer, is anxious, and fears isolation. Despite the fact that he is a patient with cancer, he is essentially a patient and should be regarded as such. He can be irritated by hospitalization and treatments and displace this on the food and boredom. The dietitian and the occupational therapist address this and exercise their skills. Family visits should be encouraged.

The oncologist should inform his patient in a manner that is clear, unhurried, supportive, and accepting of his patient's utilization of defense mechanisms. The oncologist should not take personally his patient's dependency, demandingness, or therapeutic reclacitrancy, but rather understand that this is the patient's response to regression. In the same vein, the helpers meet the family with calmness, and a willingness to suppress personal annoyance or restlessness.

This is not to suggest that the helpers be all-accepting and permissive because this would not be in the patient's best interest. Also, because one has a life-threatening illness, does not mean that the person is suddenly holy or good. One dies as one has lived. If one has been infanitle or rigid, one will be the same during the progress of the disease. If one has been flexible in one's coping, one will do likewise with illness. In a sense, instead of "dying of cancer," one can "live with cancer." Whether one is a "good" patient or not, he remains a patient as well as a human. This dictates that he be treated with concerned respect and appropriate therapy.[32]

As time and treatments unfold, issues arise. Early on, physical and emotional complications such as infections, pain, body image changes, depression, and more develop and continue. The providers are not without resources. There are medications to combat infections and alleviate pain, tranquilizers for anxiety, and antidepressants when appropriate. Of course, requests for visits from clergy or lawyers are granted and, at times, even encouraged.

Most useful to the patient are his human contacts: family, friends, and helpers of all levels. Also, his use of denial. Denial equates with *hope,* and as such is crucial to his acceptance of therapy and all of its potentially humiliating and painful side effects. To blatantly attack the use of denial is to deprive the patient of hope. Hope can be realistic; insulin and the poliomyelitis vaccine give testimony to this fact. The skillful helpers will walk the thin line between repeatedly and consistently directing the patient toward reality and at the same time, permitting the patient the integrity of his denial. If there is insistence on reality, the patient will lose all hope. The overemphasis on denial leaves the patient feeling inadequate to deal with his illness and the demands he must meet.

Finally, there is the grieving, by the patient and his family. This process begins with diagnosis and continues throughout the illness and the helpers intervene only when necessary, ie, if the relatives are functioning against the patient's best interests.

During the course of the patient's illness, and even at the end, the helpers *listen.* Listening is an art which is tedious and, at times, difficult. But where cure is not possible, suffering can be ameliorated. By listening, the helpers permit the patient to ventilate about anything and everything, personal and/or seemingly inconsequential matters. Families should also be encouraged to listen to their ill relative. There are "death and dying" savants who advocate that families press the patient to discuss his "feelings" about his death. Most patients will discuss their thoughts and feelings about death (usually intellectualized-denial) with their helpers. But not so with their families, for patients fear they would experience guilt for further "burdening" the family with their illness.

The theme of the plot in the cancer drama is the relationship of humans to humans. Not the medical-biological model, nor the intellectualized social psychological philosophical model. Both models are important for the helpers' understanding of this difficult area and insight into one's own feelings. But before the curtain falls, the protagonist, the cancer patient, needs calm, unfrightened, warm human contact from the other actors in the play. Whether the performance is on the stage of living or the stage of dying, the roles are equally arduous. A successful passage through both provides the entire cast with a gratifying sense of accomplishment.

REFERENCES

1. N. Schnaper, Postanesthetic (postoperative) emotional responses. Anesthesiology, 22:674-81, 1961.
2. J. E. Finesinger, H. C. Shands, and R. D. Abrams, Managing the emotional problems of the cancer patient. In *Clinical Problems in Cancer Research.* New York: American Cancer Society, 1952, 106-121.
3. J. E. Finesinger, S. Cobb, and R. D. Abrams, Psychological mechanisms in patients with cancer. *Cancer, 4:*1159-70, 1951.
4. R. D. Abrams and J. E. Finesinger, Guilt reactions in patients with cancer. *Cancer, 6:*474-82, 1953.
5. E. M. Pattison, Experience of dying. *Am J Psychother, 21:*32-43, 1967.
6. H. Feifel (Ed.), *The Meaning of Death.* New York: McGraw-Hill, 1977.
7. R. Fulton, *Death and Identity.* New York: John Wiley & Sons, 1965.
8. B. G. Glaser and A. Straus, *Awareness of Dying.* Chicago: Aldine, 1966.
9. R. Kastenbaum, *Death, Society and Human Experience.* St. Louis: C. V. Mosby, 1977
10. N. Schnaper, Emotional responses of the surgical patient. in Tice's *Practice of Medicine,* vol. 10. Hagerstown, MD: Harper & Row, 1969, chap. 44, pp.1-14.
11. G. Gorer, *Death, Grief and Mourning in Contemporary Britain.* London: Cresset Press, 1965.

12. C. M. Parkes, *Bereavement: Studies of Grief in Adult Life.* New York: Columbia University Press, 1975.
13. B. Schoenberg et al., *Bereavement: Its Psychosocial Aspects.* New York: Columbia University Press, 1975.
14. S. Freud, *Mourning and Melancholia: Collected Papers,* vol. 4. London: Hogarth Press, 1917.
15. N. Schnaper, Management of the dying patient. In E. T. Lisansky and B. Shochet (Eds.), *Modern Treatment,* Hagerstown, Md: Harper & Row, 1969, pp. 749-59.
16. N. Schnaper, What preanesthetic visit? *Anesthesiology. 22:*486-88, 1961.
17. N. Schnaper, "Down the tube?" No: "resource"—the language of oncology. *New Engl J Med, 296:*883, 1972.
18. Z. J. Lipowski, Consultation—liaison psychiatry: an overview, *Am J Psychiatry, 131:*623-30, 1974.
19. N. Schnaper and R. A. Growley, Overview: psychiatric sequelae to multiple trauma, *Am J Psychiatry. 133:8,* 1976.
20. A. D. Weisman, Death and responsibility: a psychiatrist's view. *Psychiatr Opinion, 3:*22-26, 1966.
21. M. I. Donovan and S. G. Pierce, *Cancer Care Nursing.* New York: Appleton Century-Crofts, 1976.
22. E. A. Smith, *Psychological Aspects of Cancer Patient Care.* New York: McGraw Hill, 1975.
23. E. A. Smith, *A Comprehensive Approach to Rehabilitation of the Cancer Patient.* New York: McGraw-Hill, 1976.
24. M. H. Browning and E. P. Lewis, *Nursing and the Cancer Patient: A Compilation of Articles from* American Journal of Nursing, Nursing Research, and Nursing Outlook. New York: American Journal of Nursing Company, 1973.
25. J. Eaton, Coping with staff grief. In *Nurse as Care-Giver for the Terminal Patient and His Family.* New York: Columbia University Press, 1976, pp.140-45.
26. R. D. Abrams, The responsibility of social work in terminal cancer. In B. Schoenberg, A. C. Carr, D. Peretz, and A. H. Kutscher (Eds.), *Psychosocial Aspects of Terminal Care.* New York: Columbia University Press, 1972, pp. 173-82.
27. M. A. Rose, Problems families face. *Am J Nurs, 76:*416-18, 1976.
28. B. L. Harker, Cancer and communication problems: a personal experience. *Psychiatr Med, 3:*163-71, 1972.
29. R. D. Abrams, The patient with cancer—his changing patterns of communication. *New Engl J Med, 274:*317-22, 1966.
30. L. Leiber et al., The communication of affection between cancer patients and their spouses. *Psychosom Med, 38:*379-89, 1976.
31. R. D. Abrams, Social casework with cancer patients. *Social Casework, 32:*425-32, 1951.
32. N. Schnaper, Death and dying: has the topic been beaten to death? *J Nerv Ment Dis, 160:*157-8, 1975.

Chapter 15

SUDDEN DEATH IN THE EMERGENCY DEPARTMENT: A COMPREHENSIVE APPROACH FOR FAMILIES, EMERGENCY MEDICAL TECHNICIANS, AND EMERGENCY DEPARTMENT STAFF

STEPHEN M. SOREFF

Sometimes death leaps suddenly upon its victims like a thug.
Robert Louis Stevenson

Death in the Emergency Department (ED) requires a comprehensive approach with attention and sensitivity to families,[1,3] Emergency Medical Technicians (EMT), ED staff and house officers. When the patient dies, the staff still has a responsibility to help the family. Furthermore, staff can help themselves, their students, and their house officers deal with these deaths.

Several significant features distinguish a patient's death in the ED from a patient's expiration in the hospital. First, the death happens suddenly and unexpectedly. No one foresaw the automobile accident or the heart attack. The resultant death came without warning. For the hospitalized individual, he himself, his family and the staff often anticipate the end and attempt to prepare for it.[3] Second, the patient and his family frequently do not know ED staff before the event. Commonly, staff must locate, telephone, and then request the family to come to the ED. There,

Stephen M. Soreff, Sudden Death in the Emergency Department: A Comprehensive Approach for Families, Emergency Medical Technicians, and Emergency Department Staff, *Critical Care Medicine*, 7:321-3. Copyright 1979, The Williams & Wilkins Co. Reproduced by permission.

staff and family meet for the first time. In contrast, the hospital-ized patient has a chart and relationship with the staff. His family has met, talked, and worked with doctors and nurses. Third, the ED death not infrequently represents the first time a medical student, a house officer, or nursing student will encounter the loss of one of his patients. All these characteristics make it mandatory to prepare for the unexpected sudden death.

The comprehensive approach to sudden death in the ED must include and take into account an effective telephone technique, the availability of a private room, staff-family interactions, the physician's encounters with the family, their reactions to the death, their confrontation with the body, the chaplain's role, the staff's reactions, the EMTs responses, and the student's experi-ences.

The telephone provides the ED staff with a major treatment modality. They can use it to help identify the patient, to secure valuable information, to locate the family, and to gain their attendance in the ED. But the telephone activity requires staff to employ proper techniques. In all ED telephone contacts, staff must first identify themselves. Then, whenever possible, the staff should not inform the family of the death over the telephone, but rather have them come to the ED; the staff also might suggest a friend drive the family member to the ED. Physicians often can recall informing a family member over the telephone of a patient's death, followed by the relative responding with "Oh my God!" and hanging up. Subsequent calls are met by either a busy signal or no answer and the physician is left perplexed and concerned.

A quiet office with a telephone, out of the main activity of the ED, offers the family a measure of dignity and privacy in the midst of the crisis. The family finds staying in the waiting room or pacing the corridor outside a trauma room uncomfortable and disquieting. In those places, they are disturbed, terrified, and overwhelmed by the activity they observe and by the fragments of conversations they overhear. This office also gives the physicians and nurses an opportunity to talk with the family privately without interruptions and distractions. The family can use the room as a place to receive friends and relatives, or just to cry. Finally, the telephone permits the family to make the important calls to relatives, friends, clergy, and a funeral home.

The ED staff plays a critical role in how the family relates to the events. Staff has a particularly great responsibility towards the family and they must monitor their statements and expressions because the family weighs for months the words and responses of the staff and reviews for a lifetime the happenings of that day. When the family is present before the patient's death, the staff can help families. Frequent staff meetings should be held with the family during the treatment. This not only keeps the family informed of the ED efforts, but provides a way for staff to work with the family. The family appreciates knowing what is being done for their loved one.

The ED physician has the responsibility of telling the family of the patient's death. Although frequently he is not their family doctor and he may not have the advantage of a prior relationship, he can be of great comfort to the family. First, he helps by frequent contacts with the family during the treatment. Second, he tells them of the death in a private office when they are seated. Third, he informs them of the treatment rendered. The family appreciates knowing everything possible was done for their loved one. Fourth, he accompanies them to see the body. Finally, he spends a few minutes with them, just listening, just being with them.

The family experiences acute grief upon hearing of the death; a flood of emotions and questions engulf them.[4] Many emerge stunned by the death. One mother whose 6-month old son was pronounced dead in the ED with the diagnosis of Sudden Infant Death Syndrome reported feeling "numb" for a month. They recoil with anger, tears, sadness, helplessness, despair, and disbelief. Their world has been shattered. Feelings of guilt and blame overwhelm them. They meticulously review recent events to find a cause and search for a reason for the unreasonable. In their quest for an answer, they can be hardest upon themselves. Had they left the child unattended? Had they fought with the spouse before the heart attack? Had they ignored his physical complaints? Had they driven the car improperly? The family confronts a series of painful emotions which they neither had anticipated nor were prepared for.

Staff have a particularly difficult task in their responsibility concerning the family's sense of guilt. On one hand, they must make appropriate inquiry of the family to determine the circumstances of the accident or to derive information concerning the medical emergency. On the other hand, family often views such questions as accusations. Again, in the case of an unexpected infant death, when staff are asked how long the child has been alone and if the baby had had a cold, the mother may perceive this as an attack upon her and her parenting ability; she may feel guilty.[5] All staff interactions and comments will be meticulously studied and remembered by the family.

Many families wish to see their loved one's body. The sudden unexpected nature of the death explains the family's disbelief and the importance of seeing the body. The confrontation with the body helps the family to begin to integrate the loss. The family's viewing of the body gives them a chance to say "goodbye." Often ED personnel are more concerned with the anticipated reactions of the family than the family actually exhibit.

The chaplain plays a critical role. In the turbulent seas of the ED, the chaplain provides an island of calm and sustenance. Certainly, most families want their minister, priest, or rabbi, but in such emergencies, I have been impressed by the value of a supportive clergyman to the family regardless of the denominational match. A chaplain can spend that most precious of qualities with the family—time! The ED staff must attend to other duties.The chaplain stays with the family; he starts to address the unanswerable questions; he puts the family in touch with the clergy they want for the funeral and he has practical information about funerals. In fact, one chaplain strongly recommends the family make contact with a funeral home before leaving the ED.

The death affects the entire ED staff. The mood of the ED reflected the tragedy and the family's grief. Individuals feel the loss. Many struggle with the sense of failure.[6] They had been there to save lives, instead they have been confronted with their limitations. The physician had to deal with "his own disappointment with his profession and fallibility."[7]

I recommend they discuss among themselves their reaction to these cases. As a consultant psychiatrist to an ED, I participated in a series of monthly staff meetings concerning these issues.[8]

Many staff members shared intense feelings. They felt frustrated, bewildered, angry, guilty, and hopeless. They also concluded they could do more for the families. A coffee room within the ED provides an excellent place for staff to review these cases and also to discuss them with involved EMTs. Emergency medicine training programs should include a comprehensive approach to death in the ED.

The EMT reactions parallel those of the ED with two important differences. While the ED staff have come to appreciate their limitations in these cases, EMTs often have not had years of training nor such an extensive background. Additionally, EMTs, especially volunteers, often disperse after the transportation is completed. In contrast, the ED staff benefits from group support and review. For example, three volunteer rescue workers transported a 55-year old businessman with chest pain who experienced cardiac arrest in the ambulance while en route to the hospital. The patient was pronounced dead on arrival. One EMT was so overwhelmed by the death he dropped out of participation in the rescue unit. Their curriculum should include and underscore the importance of the family's reaction. They must view the family as part of their treatment and transport responsibility. They must review and discuss these cases.

Many medical students, house officers, and nursing students find an ED death particularly difficult and stressful. Little in their training prepared them for these events and the subsequent impact. For some, this will be the first death of *his* patient. It will also mark the first time he will have to tell the family of the death. One house officer vividly recalls meeting a mother and four teenagers and telling them their father died en route to the hospital. The family, literally, emotionally dissolved in front of him. He felt overwhelmed by their reaction and rapidly left the family. He was not prepared to deal with them. Some students question their role and commitment to the health professions after such deaths in the ED. A nursing student almost decided to leave school after witnessing an ED death.

Finally, staff must be particularly attentive and responsive to house officers and other students in cases of ED deaths. Appropriate empathic management of the family by the physician provides an excellent model for which house officers can identify.

Medical, nursing, and physician assistants school curriculum and house officer training should include management of ED deaths.

REFERENCES

1. R. L. Stevenson, Aes Triples. In *Viginibus Puerisque and Other Essays in Belle Lettres.* London: William Heinemann, 1924.
2. E. S. Shneidman, *Deaths of Man.* New York: Macmillan, 1970.
3. E. Kubler-Ross, *On Death and Dying.* New York: Macmillan, 1970.
4. E. Lindemann, Symptomatology and management of acute grief. *Am J Psychiatry, 101:*141, 1944.
5. S. E. Weinstein, Sudden Infant Syndrome: impact on families and a direction for change. *Am J Psychiatry, 135:*831, 1978.
6. D. Hendin, *Death as a Fact of Life.* New York: W. W. Norton, 1973.
7. J. Spikes and J. Holland, The physician's response to the dying patient. In J. J. Strain and S. Grossman (Eds.), *Psychological Care of the Medically Ill.* New York: Appleton-Century-Crofts, 1975.
8. S. Soreff, Psychiatric consultation in the emergency department. *Psychiatric Ann, 8:*4, 1978.

Chapter 16

SUMMARY

George Henderson

_____

The overarching element of the physician-patient communication process is empathy. Patients are influenced to follow a medical regimen when their physicians project empathic credibility. Whether they come of their own free will or are coerced, most patients enter the medical arena with preconceived notions of what is interpersonally satisfying. Consequently, unless the physician is able to establish rapport with the patient, much of his/her medical skills will be unused or inappropriately used.

THE COMMUNICATION PROCESS

By the very nature of their training and professional vow, all physicians should be concerned with helping patients. However, helping is a complex task that requires an understanding of human communication. Verbal and nonverbal communication are integral parts in both the definition and treatment of illnesses.

> Verbal and nonverbal influences interact in ways previously unsuspected in processes intimately involved in illnesses. The study of this interaction discloses the profound effect of the two signalling systems in the life of feeling and of bodily processes, normal and pathlogical. Ulcers of the stomach seem clear manifestations of illness; tears and blushing are not so named. The second signalling system, verbal processes, regulates bodily functions, as when someone weeps in recounting a loss. The name "illness," on the other hand, poorly differentiates ulcers from tears: This is one of the many errors of the symbolic process.[1]

The Context of Physician-Patient Communication

Communication constitutes the basic process of human inter-

189

action. Most definitions of human communication include explicit or implicit references to a dynamic, irreversible process. Equally important, it is a symbolic process that allows humans to transcend their physical limitations. That is, through communication (symbolic interaction) humans are able to recall their past, analyze their present, and predict their future. Without symbolization each of us would be trapped in our own skin, unable to communicate our personal experiences to others. Through communication, illnesses are described, cures are discovered, and rehabilitation plans are devised.

Usually, the patient must send the first message in a physician-patient communication: "Help me, I'm sick." Most people are hesitant to admit they are sick, and it is only after being told that they are by their significant other persons do they adopt the patient role. Sickness implies exemption from normal social role responsibilities, a condition that must be changed, a desire to get well, and an obligation to cooperate with the physician. There are many factors that provide a context for physician-patient communication, including environment, culture, social roles, and power relationships.

ENVIRONMENT. We need only to look around us in order to see how the physical environment affects the quality of the physician-patient interaction. For example, consider the differences between an inner city slum and an affluent suburb, mountains and seashores, chemically polluted and nonpolluted communities. Environments are equivalent to nonverbal statements about health care—they cause physicians and patients to feel fearful or relaxed, cheerful or sad, claustrophobic or free.

CULTURE. Culture preference or bias is a major problem in physician-patient interacton. Members of different cultures not only speak different languages, they also live in different worlds. Inability to understand and communicate with culturally different people will render physicians unable to be optimally effective treating all patients.

SOCIAL ROLES. Shakespeare said it very well in *As You Like It:* "All the world's a stage/ And all men and women merely players./ They have their exits and their entrances,/ And one man in his time plays many parts." Some individuals forget that "physician" is a role and not themselves. Conversely, "patient" is a role and not the essence of the individual so labeled. Inflexible role players are unable to change when situations require role adaptation.

POWER. It is no secret that physicians have power over patients. Physicians who are authoritarian and dominating tend to be less helpful than their colleagues who are democratic and encourage patient initiative. Most physician messages to patients follow the classic power flow interaction process: (1) communication flows more readily laterally between physicians or between patients than either downward from physicians to patients or upward from patients to physicians, (2) more communication goes from physicians to patients than from patients to physicians, (3) patients are more cautious than physicians about the messages they send, (4) physicians and patients incorrectly assume the extent they are being understood by each other, (5) patients distort the messages they receive from physicians, and (6) both physicians and patients tend to avoid talking to each other.

Part of the physician's dilemma is that he/she must be sufficiently detached from patients to exercise sound judgment and at the same time have enough concern for patients to provide sensitive, empathic care. It is possible for a physician to suppress on the conscious level emotional responses while exploring and cutting on patients, but this detachment does not remove the stress and concern hidden in the unconscious domain of the mind. The pathological process of detachment which tends to produce mature physicians also tends to produce cynical clinicians.

Barriers Impeding Communication

Negative attitudes, stereotypes, and prejudices are three major barriers impeding physician-patient communication. Simply stated, attitudes are psychological states that predispose individuals to behave in a given manner when they encounter a specific object or situation. Stereotypes are attitudinal sets in which an individual assigns positive or negative attributes to another person on the basis of the category or group to which he/she belongs. For example, stereotyping might lead a physician to believe that all terminal patients fear death. Or, a male physician might believe that all women are hypochondriacs.

Prejudices are attitudinal sets that predispose individuals to behave in certain ways toward people solely because of their group membership. For example, females may believe that all male physicians are sexist and therefore reject male advice. The major source of physician-patient communication problems is *ethnocentrism*, the belief that one's group is superior to all others. We can readily see examples of ethnocentrism during the periods when black physicians were denied membership in the American Medical Association and women were denied admission to medical schools. In both instances, the in-group believed they were superior to the out-group. Many physicians believe they are superior to nonphysicians.

The key point in these illustrations is that *behavior*, not attitudes or beliefs, comprise the major physician-patient problem. There are many laws against discriminatory behavior, but there are none outlawing attitudes and beliefs. Patient rights advocates are quick to point out that it is what physicians *do*, not what they think about patients, that hurts or helps. Much of the interaction characterizing physician-patient communication is dehumanizing. Dehumanization is the process of perceiving oneself or others as essentially subhuman. Both the victims and the perpetrators of this cruel hoax make scientific medicine a barbaric activity.

There is a growing body of literature in medical journals that points out the importance of language differences between cultural groups. It is erroneous to assume that an interpreter is all that is needed to facilitate communication. Language and culture are inseparably bound together, and it is impossible to fully understand one without understanding the other. Physicians who understand the physiology of the body but not the psychodynamics of culture are only half-prepared to interpret medical histories.

The patient's ability to communicate his/her symptoms is an important aspect of medical diagnosis. Because they are subjective in the sense that the patient feels the symptoms and the physician does not, it is difficult for physicians to accurately interpret a patient's message. Some symptoms are ambiguous and typical of more than one condition. Besides, the etiology of physical and mental disorders are culturally influenced. Pain, for example, has varying levels of cultural definition. Some cultural groups loudly complain about pain at the first instance, while other groups believe pain is to be endured and complained about only when it becomes unbearable. Furthermore, it is not always easy to distinguish between illnesses which are psychogenic and those physiologic in origin.

Studies of physicians who are effective communicating with patients suggest that, like Abraham H. Maslow's self-actualized people, they have few ego centered thoughts during a medical interview. Their attention is focused on the patient. Methodologically, their major effort centers on collecting data and correctly understanding it. The first rule of communication is that physicians should understand their patients' values. The second rule is that physicians should adapt their communicative behavior to their patient's value systems. This implies respect for different cultural values, but it does not mean physicians should "talk down" to patients. As transmitters of messages to patients, physicians should—

1. Use simple, accurate words to describe their diagnoses and treatment plans.
2. Provide patients with enough information so that they can put the message into proper perspectives.
3. Secure validation of what patients understand.
4. Clarify the nature of their statements so that facts, beliefs, opinions, and assumptions are clearly delineated.

As receivers of messages from patients, physicians should—

1. Receive the messages with open minds.
2. Listen, read, or observe the entire communication.
3. Seek clarification of ambiguous messages.
4. Validate asserted facts and seek missing information.

Physicians walk a thin line, of which they all fall off at some time. The public expects—and frequently gets—medical science miracles. The communication task is formidable: patients must be given the best chance of getting well and the least chance of disillusionment. This, of course, is the perennial problem of humanely managing the living, consoling the dying, and giving dignity to the dead. Clearly, considerable human relations skills are needed to perform these tasks. The physician's role in the therapeutic relationship evolves around technical skills, impartiality, and the ability to communicate with patients. In our imperfect world we tend to expect perfection from individuals to whom we entrust our lives.

A DELICATE RELATIONSHIP

The physician-patient relationship necessarily is based on acceptance, expectation, support, and stimulation.[2] "Acceptance" means to unconditionally give oneself to and to receive another person. The clinician accepting a patient is communicating "I will apply my medical knowledge to help you and, as I do this, I will try to meet your needs, try to understand you, and try to respect your right to retain your own identity." In most instances, these nurturing qualities are not easily taught or freely applied. Yet, the ability to accept a patient is the *sine qua non* of the helping relationship.

"Expectation" means the projection that responsive behavior will occur. Physicians expect their patients to follow the health plan, while patients expect their physicians to devise the best possible health plan for them. Usually, physicians are quite explicit and direct in their expectations. Patients tend to be less direct and to rely more on nonverbal behavior to express themselves.

For some physicians the support and stimulus needed to continue treating a patient comes from positive rehabilitation. For others it comes from fees received. For yet others it is a combination of rehabilitation and fees. Patients, on the other hand, tend to receive their support and stimulus from positive rehabilitation and interpersonal relationships mainly with family members.

The more effective physicians are able to project to a patient an image of genuine concern, empathy, and technical skill. Even this may not be sufficient to dissolve a patient's fears and anxieties. There is something inherently disconcerting about having to seek professional medical help. Although talking may not allay a patient's fears and anxieties, it can certainly pave the way for this to occur. Most frequently the patient will begin the initial medical interview by telling the physician what he/she thinks the problem to be. However, there are many instances when a patient will remain silent or inarticulate or talk about nonrelated issues. As the patient or a spokesperson tells his/her symptoms, glibly or haltingly, the physician should communicate that he/she not only understands but also empathizes. Failure to do this will result in the termination of the relationship.

> Ethnocentrism makes it difficult for providers to communicate with many minority patients. And lack of awareness of a patient's cultural preferences and style of interaction often generates antagonisms which lead to curtailed or aborted treatment. A classic example is found in a confrontation between an Anglo physician and a traditional South Texas Chicano. After the physician laughed at the Chicano's diagnosis that his wife's complaint resulted from witchcraft, the physician ordered the lady to undress. "This I could not stand, that my wife should be naked with this man. We never returned, of course, and my wife was treated by a folk healer. Maybe Anglos let doctors stare at their wives' bodies and fool around with them, but not me. And the fool didn't even know about *susto* [magically induced fright]. He is lucky I did not reduce his arrogance right there."[3]

Patients tend to take their cues from physicians. Insensitivity to a patient's belief and fears may result in premature termination of the consultation. Most patients need time to talk, to listen, and to learn about scientific medical beliefs and practices. Relatedly, to tell patients and their relatives not to be embarrassed or feel guilty because they do not fully understand an illness may inadvertently suggest that they *should* experience these feelings.

When feelings are expressed and received the distance between physician and patient is spanned. As the physician-patient relationship unfolds, the scientific background of the physician comes to the center of the interaction. Both verbally and nonverbally, an effective physician will communicate expertise. For most patients this means becoming exposed to new ways of defining and treating their health problems. Unfortunately, new ways are not always easy to accept.

It is important for the physician to explain the technical aspects of disease and illness in terms that will make treatment procedures rational to lay persons. Research data show that if patients are to willingly and accurately follow a medical regimen, they must understand and accept the physician's diagnoses and treatment plans. This is a basic human relations principle: *individuals affected by a plan must understand it if optimum compliance is to occur.*

When the patient is nourished and sustained by contact with the physician, the relationship is not only good but also helpful. Medical students would do well to remember that most patients are like the Philosopher in James Stephens' *The Crock of Gold*, who said, "I have learned that the head does not hear anything until the heart has listened, and that what the heart knows today the head will understand tomorrow."[4]

Physicians have feelings, too, and part of their professional skill is the management of them. Physicians have feelings of likes and dislikes, happiness and grief, security and insecurity, competence and imcompetence. They may be strongly attracted to some patients and repelled by others. They respond to patients with feeling. The challenge is to minimize unfair, nonprofessional treatment and to maximize fair, professional treatment of *all* patients.

HELPING PATIENTS TO COMMUNICATE

Helping patients to tell what ails them requires more than a receptive listener. Physicians who believe that the structured interview is the only effective method of eliciting pertinent data should learn from the experiences of social workers.

> It has long been said in casework, reiterated against the sometime practice of subjecting the client to a barrage of ready-made questions, that the client "should be allowed to tell his story in his own way." Particularly at the beginning this is true, because the client may feel an urgency to do just that, to pour out what *he* sees and thinks and feels because it is his problem and because he has lived with it and mulled it within himself for days or perhaps months. Moreover, it is "his own way" that gives both caseworker and client not just the objective facts of the problem, but the grasp of its significance. To the client who is ready and able to "give out" with what troubles him, the caseworker's nods and murmurs of understanding—any of those nonverbal ways by which we indicate response—may be all the client needs in his first experience of telling and being heard out.[5]

Not all patients can easily talk about themselves and their illnesses. Comments such as "I can imagine that this is not easy for you to talk about" or "Go on, I'm listening" may be enough encouragement for some reticent patients. Others will need direct questions to help them focus their conversation. One of the most difficult and important professional helper roles is that of listener. A good case history is not the result of passive listening:

it is the by-product of manipulative and interpretive talking and active listening. Effective listening is demanding; most physicians have to work hard at listening to what the patient is trying to say.

Few people know exactly what is ailing them until they have communicated sufficient data to a physician or other medical personnel. To tell medical personnel what they are feeling is in itself a relief for many patients. But telling is not enough. Cure or rehabilitation must follow if the patient is to continue the relationship. This is likely to occur when the physician's and the patient's questions pertaining to the illness are answered. Typical patient questions include the following:

1. What is wrong with me?
2. Am I normal?
3. What caused it?
4. What's going to happen to me?
5. What can I do to help?

The words of Paul Tournier sum up the process of helping patients to communicate, "Through information I can understand a case, only through communication shall I be able to understand a person...."[6] The dynamics of health care are threefold. (1) The facts that constitute the health problem must be understood. Facts frequently consist of objective reality and subjective reactions. (2) The facts must be thought through. They must be probed into, reorganized, and turned over in order for the physician to grasp as much of the total configuration as possible. (3) A plan must be devised that will result in resolving or alleviating the problem. While an ideal, suffering cannot always be eliminated.

> Certainly we always try to eliminate suffering and especially pain. But it is not the task of therapy merely to reduce mental and physical suffering. One may be inclined to do this because one assumes that the elimination of suffering is an essential or even *the* essential drive of man, as psychoanalysis proclaims in the form of pleasure principle. But placing this in the foreground would often *not* help the patient. The idea of the pleasure principle, particularly when applied to normal life, overlooks the enormous significance of tension for self-realization in its highest form. Pleasure, in the sense of relief from tension, may be a necessary state of respite. But it is a phenomenon of "stand still".... One can achieve the right attitude toward the problem of the elimination of suffering in patients and in normal individuals

only if one considers the significance for self-realization and its relationship to the value of health. If the patient is able to make the choice we may have mentioned he may still suffer, but may *no longer feel sick*, i.e., though somewhat disordered and stricken by a certain anxiety, he is able to realize his essential capacities at least to a considerable degree.[7]

According to Daniel M. Laskin, this type of "verbal 'sedation' can be as effective as pharmacologic sedation. Such an effort not only makes the entire experience more acceptable, but also reduces the possibility of stress-related medical complications."[8] However, we should not view communication as a placebo component of treatment. An accurate diagnosis and a proper treatment plan are essential to the physician-patient relationship.

A health problem cannot be solved if the necessary resources are missing. Here, again, communication is a key factor. Like any puzzle, missing pieces of information in a health problem will render it insolvable. But information alone is seldom enough. And too much information can freeze negative attitudes. Thus, the decision about how much information to give a patient should not be made lightly.

Before and after giving a patient information, the physician should ask the patient if he/she has any questions. It is common for physicians (and other health care professionals) to give instructions that are nonspecific, incomplete, and inexplicable. For example, consider the vagueness of written instructions to take medicine "as directed" or "one tablet three times a day." In the latter case, should the medicine be taken every eight hours or with meals? Medical communication has three broad objectives:

1. *Surveillance*—helping the patient to detect that the drug is improving his condition, to detect side effects of the drug, to monitor other changes in health, etc.
2. *Correlation*—helping the patient to organize a set of procedures (we organize, but the patient has to carry them out), helping the patient to get along in the health care environment, etc.
3. *Education*—helping the patient to understand the whys behind his treatment and/or disease.[9]

Most patients—especially those in traditional folk cultures—need to learn how to explore new and contradictory health ideas and facts. The greater the cultural distance between patients and orthodox medicine, the more likely medical advice will be misunderstood or ignored. Frequently, patients want to change their health habits but do not know how or feel too threatened by the thought of change. Finally, physicians should focus their medical probing on problems that can be resolved within the health-care setting. For example, while it may be interesting to learn the political views of a patient, this information will do little to relieve her arthritis.

WHY BOTHER

The problems of physician-patient communication are more complex than many authors suggest. Seldom is a physician taught to elicit information—how to talk, to listen, and to provide feedback. But this is not to suggest that there are no physicians who can effectively communicate with patients. There are many who possess this skill. However, most of them are self-taught. Something as important as communication should not be left to intuition or chance. Nor should the patient's understanding the physician be left to chance.

Numerous studies conclude that a large number of patients receive insufficient information about their conditions and treatment. Specifically, many patients are released from treatment without ever having understood what their physician diagnosed as their illness, why certain procedures were followed, and—if operated upon—what their operation consisted of and the reasons for the related preparations. The patient's rights include the right to courteous, prompt, and the best treatment; and the right to know what is wrong, why, and what is going to be done about it.

We could build a case of patient ignorance as being a by-product of the medical mystique. That is, scientific medicine is commonly perceived as being administered by men and women whose training and predilections place them in a special service category. To put it even more bluntly, there is a tendency for patients to be in awe of physicians. But beyond this intangible dimension of the physician-patient communication process, physicians remain divided over what information should be given to patients and how information should be given.

There are many reasons for physician failure to communicate pertinent information to patients. Some physicians make no effort to communicate to patients information about their illness. In other instances, patients fail to request information, particularly that which would give them basic understanding of their illness. Since human communication is a two-way process, both physicians and patients distort messages. Some patients forget medical information that had been clearly communicated to them. This sheds doubt on the validity of respondent dissatisfaction with the medical information they have received. Furthermore research is sparse that demonstrates that patients who understand their illness get well faster than those who do not. From this narrow perspective, we could conclude that patients' understanding of their illness in unimportant if adequate histories can be obtained and patients follow prescribed treatment. However, if the goals of medicine include relieving, reassuring, and restoring patients, then it is important for patients to understand their illness.

It is likely that patients who are the most confused about their condition and what their physicians are doing are less actively involved in discussions with physicians than patients who are better informed. Unfortunately, most physicians cannot accurately judge the level of their patients' medical knowledge. An old adage seems appropriate: when in doubt, ask. There are several ways the more effective physicians communicate with patients and their relatives. Some physicians verbally tell their patients the information; others use printed materials, including diagrams and leaflets. Still others refer patients to commercial audiovisual material. In the end, the quality of the information a physician is able to give a patient is directly related to the quality of information he/she gets from the patient.

REFERENCES

1. William C. Lewis, *Why People Change: The Psychology of Influence.* New York: Hold, Rinehard & Winston, 1972, p. 224.
2. Helen Harris Perlman, *Social Casework: A Problem-solving Process.* Chicago: University of Chicago Press, 1957, pp. 67-83.
3. Jerry L. Weaver and Sharon D. Garrett, Sexism and racism in the American health industry: a comparative analysis. *Internat J Health Care,* 8:697, 1978.

4. James Stephens, *The Crock of Gold*. New York: Macmillan, 1946, p. 128.
5. Perlman, *op.cit.*, p. 142.
6. Paul Tournier, *The Meaning of Persons*. New York: Harper & Row, 1957, p. 25.
7. Kurt Goldstein, Health as a value. In Abraham H. Maslow (Ed.), *New Knowledge in Human Values*. Chicago: Henry Regnery, 1959, pp. 182-3.
8. Daniel M. Laskin, Doctor-patient relationship: a potential communication gap. *J Oral Surg*, 37:786, 1979.
9. Marianne Ivey, Yvonne Tso, and Keith Stamm, Communication techniques for patient instruction. *Am J Hosp Pharm*, 32:830, 1975.

ADDITIONAL READINGS

R. Bandler and J. Grinder. *The Structure of Magic: A Book About Language and Therapy*. Palo Alto, CA: Science & Behavior Books, 1975.

I. Barofsky, Compliance, adherence and the therapeutic alliance: steps in the development of self-care. *Soc Sci Med, 12:*369-76, 1978.

G. R. Beaton, Treatment of hypertension. *S Afr Med J, 14:* 997-1000, 1978.

M. A. Benarde and E. W. Mayerson, Patient-physician negotiation. *JAMA, 239:*1413-5, 1978.

R. Berni and H. Ready. *Problem-Oriented Medical Record Implementation: Allied Health Peer Review*. St. Louis: C. V. Mosby, 1974.

P. Boreham and D. Gibson. The information process in private medical consultations: a preliminary investigation. *Soc Sci Med, 12:*409-16, 1978.

D. S. Brady, Feedback from patients as a means of teaching non-technological aspects of medical care. *J Med Educ, 55:*34-41, 1980.

————. An analysis of patient recall of their therapeutic regimens. *J Chronic Dis, 33:*57-63, 1980.

E. L. Brown, *Newer Dimensions of Patient Care*. New York: Russell Sage Foundation, 1965.

M. B. Daly and B. S. Hulka. Talking with the doctor: II. *J Commun, 25:*148-52, 1975.

L. M. Daniels and M. S. Kochas. What influences adherence to hypertension therapy. *Nurs Forum, 18:*231-45, 1979.

H. F. Dowling and T. Jones. *That the Patient May Know: An*

Atlas for Use in Explaining to the Patient. Philadelphia: Saunders, 1959.

A. Enelow and S. N. Swisher. *Interviewing and Patient Care.* New York: Oxford University Press, 1979.

H. W. Griffith, *Instruction for Patients.* Philadelphia: Saunders, 1975.

R. Hall, Helping patients take their medicare. *Aust Fam Physician, 8:*1081-5, 1979.

H. H. Hatasaka, Informed consent—defense orthodontics. *Am J Orthod, 76:*448-55, 1979.

M. Haug, Doctor-patient relationships and the older patient. *J Gerontol, 34:*852-60, 1979.

L. L. Havens, Taking a history from the difficult patient. *Lancet, 21:*138-40, 1978.

D. E. Hayes-Bautista, Modifying the treatment: patient control medical care. *Soc Sci Med, 10:*223-8, 1976.

R. M. Herbertt and J. M. Innes, Familiarization and preparatory information in the reduction of anxiety in child dental patients. *ASDC J Dent Child, 46:*319-23, 1979.

A. L. Hernandez, When the patient "won't hear of it." *Dent Manage, 19:*45-6, 1979.

A. Himmelhoch, Patient adherence in the treatment of hypertension. *Aust Fam Physician, 9:*229-34, 1980.

M. Jellinek, Referrals from a psychiatric emergency room: relationship of compliance to demographic and interview variables. *Am J Psychiatry, 135:*209-13, 1978.

S. S. Johnson, Health beliefs of hypertensive patients in a family medicine residency program *J Fam Pract, 9:*877-83, 1979.

P. Ley, Memory for medical information. *Br J Soc Clin Psychol,* 18:245-55, 1979.

D. J. Munjack and L. J. Oziel, Resistance in the behavioral treatment of sexual dysfunctions. *J Sex Marital Ther, 4:*122-38, 1978.

J. R. Neill, The difficult patient: identification and response. *J Clin Psychiatry, 40:*209-12, 1979.

N. Putnam and J. Yager, Traction intolerance syndrome: a psychiatric complication of femoral fractures. *Int J Psychiatry Med, 8:*133-43, 1977-1978.

S. M. Radius et al., Factors influencing mothers' compliance

A

Add

Additional Readings

Additional Readings 2

Additional Readings 205

with a medication regimen for asthmatic children. *J Asthma Res, 15:*133-49, 1978.

S. J. Reiser, Refusing treatment for mental illness: historical and ethical dimensions. *Am J Psychiatry, 137:*329-31, 1980.

H. P. Roth and H. S. Caron, Accuracy of doctors' estimates and patients' statements of adherence to a drug regimen. *Clinc Pharmacol Ther, 23:*361-70, 1978.

H. L. Runyon and S. O. Krolls, Patient motivation: some implications from the behavioral sciences. *Quintessence Int, 9:* 61-65.1978.

D. O. Schmidt, Patient compliance: the effect of the doctor as a therapeutic agent. *J Fam Pract, 4:* 853-6, 1977.

J. C. Shipp, Diabetes mellitus in the adult: treatment in the office setting. *Nebr Med J, 64*358-62, 1979.

B. Starfield et al., Presence of observers at patient-practitioner interactions: impact on coordination of care and methodologic implications. *Am J Public Health, 69:*102-5, 1979.

D. R. Talkington, Maximizing patient compliance by shaping attitudes of self-directed health care. *J Fam Pract, 6:*591-5, 1978.

S. Vaisrub, Helpful hate. *JAMA, 241:*1157, 1979.

S. B. Van Camerik, Why don't patients do what you tell them? *Leg Aspects Med Pract, 6:*30-33, 1978.

M. Wexler and L. M. Adler, *Help the Patient Tell His Story,* Oradell, NJ: Medical Economics, 1971.

M. Z. Wile et al. Physician-patient communication: interpretations of non-technical phrases. *Annu Conf Res Med Educ, 18:* 208-13, 1979.

F. R. Woolley et al., The effects of doctor-patient communication on satisfaction and outcome of care. *Soc Sci Med, 12:*123-8, 1978.

C. A. Wurster, P. Weinstein, and A. J. Cohen, Communication patterns in pedodontics. *Percept Mot Skills, 48:*159-66, 1979.

INDEX

Randall Library – UNCW

R727.3 .P48   NXWW
Physician–patient communication : readings and rec

304900268035/